Interdisciplinary Rheumatology

Interdisciplinary Rheumatology: Rheumatology and Gastroenterology is the first complete textbook to examine the myriad complications of rheumatic syndromes in the gastrointestinal tract. Each disease is summarized for a broad medical audience, with focus on the consequences of the disorder throughout the gut. The reader will formulate an understanding of the clinical, pharmacological, and nutritional aspects of the interface of these two specialties with expert contributors from a range of academic centers. Rheumatologists and gastroenterologists will be able to recognize, evaluate, and treat gastrointestinal symptoms of autoimmune diseases and collaborate in improving the experience and outcomes of these complex patients.

Reem Jan, MBBS BSc (Senior Editor) is a full-time academic clinical rheumatologist at the University of Chicago. She completed her medical education at St George's University of London UK, followed by an internal medicine residency and rheumatology fellowship at the University of Michigan, Ann Arbor. She has developed expertise in the diagnosis and management of complex seronegative spondyloarthritis patients. Her collaborative clinical practice includes the provision of specialist care at the University of Chicago Inflammatory Bowel Disease Center.

Sushila Dalal, MD is an academic gastroenterologist at the University of Chicago. She completed her medical education at the University of Chicago Pritzker School of Medicine, followed by an internal medicine residency and gastroenterology fellowship at the University of Chicago. She has expertise in the management of inflammatory bowel diseases.

T0313281

Interdisciplinary Rheumatology Series

For more information, please visit: https://www.routledge.com/Interdisciplinary-Rheumatology/book-series/IRJL

Interdisciplinary Rheumatology

Rheumatology and Gastroenterology

Edited by
Reem Jan and Sushila Dalal

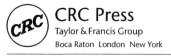

CRC Press
Taylor & Francis Group
Boca Raton London New York

CRC Press is an imprint of the
Taylor & Francis Group, an **informa** business

Designed cover image: Designed Cover

First edition published 2025
by CRC Press
2385 NW Executive Center Drive, Suite 320, Boca Raton FL 33431

and by CRC Press
4 Park Square, Milton Park, Abingdon, Oxon, OX14 4RN

CRC Press is an imprint of Taylor & Francis Group, LLC

© 2025 selection and editorial matter, Reem Jan and Sushila Dalal individual chapters, the contributors

Library of Congress Cataloging-in-Publication Data
Names: Jan, Reem, editor. | Dalal, Sushila, editor.
Title: Interdisciplinary rheumatology. Rheumatology and gastroenterology / edited by Reem Jan and Sushila Dalal.
Other titles: Rheumatology and gastroenterology | Interdisciplinary rheumatology (Series)
Description: First edition. | Boca Raton, FL : CRC Press, 2024. | Identifiers: LCCN 2024018146 (print) |
    LCCN 2024018147 (ebook) | ISBN 9781032434360 (hardback) | ISBN 9781032434353 (paperback) |
    ISBN 9781003367307 (ebook)
Subjects: MESH: Arthritis, Rheumatoid—complications | Gastrointestinal Diseases—complications |
    Arthritis, Rheumatoid—therapy | Gastrointestinal Diseases—therapy
Classification: LCC RC932 (print) | LCC RC932 (ebook) | NLM WE 346 | DDC 616.7/227—dc23/eng/20240528
LC record available at https://lccn.loc.gov/2024018146
LC ebook record available at https://lccn.loc.gov/2024018147

ISBN: 9781032434360 (hbk)
ISBN: 9781032434353 (pbk)
ISBN: 9781003367307 (ebk)

DOI: 10.1201/9781003367307

Typeset in Minion
by Apex CoVantage, LLC

Contents

Foreword

My grandmother had Crohn's disease and was diagnosed in 1954. When I started medical school at the University of Chicago in 1990, she first told me of her condition and asked me to find her a UChicago gastroenterologist and introduce myself to him as her grandson. Her doctor was Dr. Joseph B. Kirsner, a renowned clinician and patient advocate. Kirsner practiced the art of medicine and studied the science of gastrointestinal disorders for 70 years, with a special focus on the inflammatory bowel diseases (IBDs). He witnessed the IBDs emerge from an era of desperation to one in which evidence-based treatments and effective surgeries were developed, but even when I met him in 1990, there was a paucity of effective options and many people who suffered the ravages of these idiopathic conditions.

One of Kirsner's most well-read papers, "The Treatment of the 'Untreatable' Patient," was published in 1960. In this article, he emphasized the holistic care of the patient and the steadfast and meticulous devotion of the clinician to their well-being and improved quality of life and emphasis on hope for a better future, even when (especially when) medical options were not available. I have read and reread that paper multiple times. The principles of caring for the patient with chronic problems, undiagnosed conditions, and untreatable medical challenges have not changed. Nor has the importance of hope for better futures. But what I have been amazed and thankful to see change is how many conditions deemed "unknowable" or "untreatable" have been clarified and the revolutions in treatments and treatment endpoints that have changed the world for our patients. It is exactly why this edition of *Interdisciplinary Rheumatology: Rheumatology and Gastroenterology*, edited by Drs. Reem Jan and Sushila Dalal, is so necessary as a guide to these rapidly evolving diagnostic, treatment, and disease-modifying strategies.

There has been an ongoing explosion of targeted therapies for immune conditions, new insights into combination and dual-targeted treatment options, and the evolution of the science of clinical immunology, with increasing evidence and appreciation for the systemic consequences of chronic inflammation and the highly prevalent subclinical inflammation. With these advances have also emerged improved appreciation for shared pathways and the movement away from organ- or even disease-based strategies of management and toward cytokine-based approaches, dual-targeted treatments, considerations for thoughtful approaches to overlapping joint, bowel, and skin conditions, and the absolute need for multispecialty care in the management of such complex diseases. While precision medicine with therapeutic biomarkers remains in development, there are now emerged pragmatic approaches to the identification of multiorgan involvement and choice of therapies with efficacy in multiple conditions, not just to treat the multiple organ involvement with single therapeutic options but also because the existence of multiple-organ-system inflammation in an individual has implications for understanding the dominant immune pathways and targets.

I recommend this outstanding text and the unique multispecialty approach for the clinician and scientist alike. As the "untreatable" patients have become more treatable than ever, their care requires that we work together and stay abreast of the exciting and ongoing advances in our fields.

by David T. Rubin,
MD, AGAF, FACG, FACP

Citation:
Kirsner JB. The treatment of the "untreatable" patient. *Ill Med J.* 1960 Jun:117:385–400.

Preface

Hippocrates once claimed that "all diseases begin in the gut." Autoimmune diseases have long been understood to be founded on a complex interplay of genetics and environment, and in recent years, attention has turned specifically to the role of diet and the gut microbiome in the etiology of these disorders. Patients are actively involved in this quest, often looking for ways to modulate their nutrition to control inflammation and finding few reliable answers. Conversely, systemic inflammatory disorders frequently target the gastrointestinal tract, from troublesome complaints that reduce enjoyment of food to serious and life-threatening complications. This book examines the interplay between rheumatology and gastroenterology in the clinical context of major rheumatic syndromes, the pharmacology of medications used in both specialties, and the role of nutrition in the management of autoimmune diseases. It is the first complete textbook that unites the expertise of academic clinicians from both fields. We are grateful to all our authors for their contributions to this exciting project, which will allow the reader to access the most current understanding of these issues and enhance the care of patients with rheumatic disease.

Reem Jan and Sushila Dalal,
University of Chicago

Acknowledgment

We would like to thank our families for their love and support and our superb authors and collaborators from around the United States for their dedication and scholarship. We would also like to acknowledge our trainees and patients for inspiring us to reach for higher standards of knowledge and care.

Contributors

Mohamad Khaled Almujarkesh, MD
Department of Internal Medicine
Wayne State University/Detroit Medical Center
Detroit, Michigan

Nezam Altorok, MD
University of Toledo Medical Center
Division of Rheumatology
Toledo, Ohio

Shubha Bhat, PharmD, MS, BCACP
Cleveland Clinic Foundation
Cleveland, Ohio

Kevin Byram, MD
Vanderbilt University Medical Center
Department of Internal Medicine
Division of Rheumatology and Immunology
Nashville, Tennessee

Michael Cammarata, MD
Division of Rheumatology
Department of Medicine
Johns Hopkins University School of Medicine
Baltimore, Maryland

Robert Corty, MD, PhD
Vanderbilt University Medical Center
Department of Internal Medicine
Division of Rheumatology and Immunology
Nashville, Tennessee

Maya Noelle Faison, MD
University of Chicago
Chicago, Illinois

Rawish Fatima, MBBS
University of Toledo Medical Center
Division of Rheumatology
Toledo, Ohio

Jami Kinnucan, MD
Mayo Clinic Florida
Jacksonville, Florida

Kristine A. Kuhn, MD, PhD
Division of Rheumatology
University of Colorado
Anschutz Medical Campus
Denver, Colorado

Michael Macklin, MD Pharm
University of Chicago
Chicago, Illinois

Ryan Massay, MBBS (Hons)
Section of Rheumatology
University of Michigan
Ann Arbor, Michigan

Dejan Micic, MD
Section of Gastroenterology, Hepatology, and
Nutrition
University of Chicago
Chicago, Illinois

Seetha U. Monrad, MD
Section of Rheumatology
University of Michigan
Ann Arbor, Michigan

Yawen Ren, MD
Division of Rheumatology
University of Colorado
Anschutz Medical Campus
Denver, Colorado

Smarika Sapkota, MD
Division of Rheumatology
University of Colorado
Anschutz Medical Campus
Denver, Colorado

Jason Springer, MD, MS
Vanderbilt University Medical Center
Department of Internal Medicine
Division of Rheumatology and Immunology
Nashville, Tennessee

Adam C. Stein, MD
Division of Gastroenterology and Hepatology
Northwestern University
Feinberg School of Medicine
Chicago, Illinois

Chelsea Thompson, MD
Section of Rheumatology
University of Chicago
Chicago, Illinois

Kimberly Trotter, MD
Section of Rheumatology
University of Chicago
Chicago, Illinois

Approach to the Patient with Gastrointestinal Manifestations of Rheumatic Disease

SUSHILA DALAL

INTRODUCTION

Patients often come to the rheumatology clinic with multiple systemic complaints: from fatigue to poor sleep, abdominal pain, nausea, diarrhea, or bloating. Sorting out which symptoms are in the range of normal, which are medication side effects, and which are indicative of a gastrointestinal complication of rheumatic disease can be challenging. Furthermore, disorders of the gut–brain interaction, including irritable bowel syndrome, functional dyspepsia, and central abdominal pain syndrome, are prevalent in as many as 40% of the general population and can overlap with many other disorders (1). Understanding which symptoms require further testing and referral to gastroenterology is important. This chapter will review common gastrointestinal symptoms the rheumatologist may encounter, which conditions these symptoms may indicate, and further studies needed.

Diarrhea

The first step in evaluation of diarrhea is understanding what the patient means by the term "diarrhea." Important historical elements include the consistency of the stools, frequency, urgency, and the presence of blood or mucus in the stool. Understanding how long diarrhea has occurred,

whether the patient ever has formed stools, and whether diarrhea occurs at night can be helpful. Other important historical elements in the evaluation of diarrhea include possible triggers such as recent travel, sick contacts, new medications or supplements, and relationship to eating certain foods. Surgical history of bowel or gall bladder resection may also reveal causes of diarrhea. Family history of inflammatory bowel disease or celiac disease gives a higher index of suspicion for these conditions.

Acute diarrhea, or diarrhea lasting less than 14 days, is most frequently infectious. Special consideration should be given to patients with recent antibiotic use or hospitalization, who should be tested for *Clostridium difficile* infection. Patients with severe symptoms such as fever, dehydration, more than six bowel movements per day, or blood or mucus in the stool may warrant stool testing for other infections. Stool cultures test for the most common causes of infectious diarrhea: *Shigella, Salmonella, Campylobacter*, and *E. coli*. Many labs now offer a multiplexed PCR panel that tests for multiple bacterial and viral causes of diarrhea. PCR testing demonstrates that the genetic material of infectious agents is present but does not prove active infection and can have false positives. For patients on immunosuppression, consideration should also be given to infection with CMV.

DOI: 10.1201/9781003367307-1

Chronic diarrhea can be caused by inflammation, pancreatic insufficiency, surgical anatomy, medication side effects, small intestinal bacterial overgrowth, lactose intolerance, or irritable bowel syndrome. Inflammatory causes of diarrhea may be accompanied by blood or mucus in the stool, weight loss, elevated serum inflammatory markers (CRP, ESR, platelets), and decreased albumin. Calprotectin is a protein found in neutrophils. Fecal calprotectin testing can be used to distinguish between inflammatory bowel disease and irritable bowel syndrome at a cutoff of 50 ug/g (2). An elevated fecal calprotectin is suspicious for inflammatory bowel disease and should be referred for evaluation by a gastroenterologist for colonoscopy. Celiac disease can also cause diarrhea, and patients who are currently eating gluten-containing food can be tested for tissue transglutaminase IgA and deaminated gliadin IgA. Positive celiac serology testing should be referred to gastroenterology for upper endoscopy with biopsies of the duodenum.

Exocrine pancreatic insufficiency can occur in patients with chronic pancreatitis or altered pancreas anatomy. Initial screening can be accomplished with the fecal elastase test. Normal fecal elastase (> 200 mcg/g) can rule out patients with exocrine pancreatic insufficiency with low probability of disease, but low fecal elastase does result in a high false positive rate and may warrant further evaluation with pancreas imaging if a high index of suspicion exists (3).

Surgeries such as cholecystectomy or ileal resection can result in bile salt diarrhea (4). Bile salt diarrhea results from excess bile in the colon acting as an irritant to the colon lining and causing diarrhea. Bile salt diarrhea can be treated through use of bile acid sequestrant medications.

While many medications can cause diarrhea, those most relevant to the rheumatologist are NSAIDs and colchicine. Many patients often use over-the-counter magnesium supplements without realizing that magnesium is a laxative. Metformin, a commonly used diabetes medication, is also a common cause of diarrhea. Relationship of the onset of diarrhea to new medications is an important part of the history.

Lactose intolerance is common and can be suspected in cases of diarrhea that correlate with eating milk-containing foods. Testing can either be done with radiolabeled lactose breath test or with elimination of lactose from the diet. Functional diarrhea, or diarrhea not associated with an underlying structural cause, may be suspected in the absence of alarm symptoms such as weight loss, anemia, or elevated inflammatory markers. Functional diarrhea is also associated with periods of stress or anxiety and can often be accompanied by cramping or urgency. Functional diarrhea rarely occurs at night.

Dysphagia

Dysphagia refers to difficulty swallowing, while odynophagia refers to pain with swallowing. Dysphagia can occur due to esophageal strictures (often acid reflux related), cancer, eosinophilic esophagitis, web or ring, or dysmotility disorders such as achalasia or systemic sclerosis. Infection, such as with herpes simplex, *Candida*, or CMV, can cause both pain (odynophagia) and dysphagia. Initial testing should include barium esophogram if structural abnormality such as radiation, surgery, or Zenker's diverticulum is suspected. Most patients require referral to a gastroenterologist for upper endoscopy to evaluate for underlying causes of dysphagia with possible treatment with dilation when safe and feasible. If no cause for dysphagia is identified on upper endoscopy, then manometry testing for motility disorders such as those found in achalasia or systemic sclerosis can be done.

Small Intestinal Bacterial Overgrowth

Small intestinal bacterial overgrowth (SIBO) refers to GI symptoms caused by excessive bacteria in the small intestine. SIBO may be suspected in patients with bloating and diarrhea. Systemic conditions that impact gastrointestinal motility such as diabetes, systemic sclerosis, or amyloidosis are associated with increased risk of SIBO (5). Motility disorders such as pseudo-obstruction, visceral myopathies, and mitochondrial disease can also be associated with SIBO. Opiate medication use is a common cause of slow GI motility and can lead to SIBO as well. Testing can be done with glucose or lactulose hydrogen breath tests. Treatment is with an antibiotic.

Abdominal Pain

Abdominal pain can be caused a by a large variety of underlying conditions that the rheumatologist may encounter. Some of the most common causes include gastroesophageal reflux disease (GERD), dyspepsia, NSAID use with gastritis or ulcer disease, cholelithiasis or cholecystitis, pancreatitis, or gastroparesis. Constipation is also a common cause of abdominal pain. Dyspepsia refers to patients with epigastric abdominal pain, early satiety, and a sense of fullness or bloating after eating. Alarm symptoms that raise concern for malignancy and should warrant prompt referral to a gastroenterologist for evaluation with upper endoscopy include new symptoms in a patient over the age of 55, GI bleeding (melena or hematochezia), dysphagia, vomiting, unintentional weight loss, unexplained iron deficiency anemia, and family history of gastric or esophageal cancer (6). In the absence of alarm symptoms, stool or breath test for *Helicobacter pylori* with treatment eradication may be sufficient. If negative, a trial of acid-suppression medication such as PPI for H2 blocker for 4 to 8 weeks can still be beneficial. If these treatments are not effective, referral to a gastroenterologist for further evaluation and consideration of tricyclic antidepressant or prokinetic agent, depending on the patient characteristics, could be considered.

Suspicion for biliary causes of abdominal pain such as cholelithiasis or cholecystitis may be raised in patients with RUQ abdominal pain after eating a high-fat meal. Initial evaluation would include evaluation of liver function tests including bilirubin, aminotransferases, and alkaline phosphatase as well as RUQ abdominal ultrasound.

Pancreatitis may occur in response to some medications like azathioprine or 6MP or causes such as gallstones, alcohol, or elevated serum triglycerides. Evaluation for pancreatitis includes testing for lipase, which should be three times the upper limit of normal or more, and imaging with contrast-enhanced CT or MRI.

Gastroparesis may be suspected in patients with abdominal pain and bloating along with nausea and vomiting. While many cases are idiopathic, common causes also include diabetes and medications that slow motility. Evaluation of gastroparesis includes ruling out gastric outlet obstruction with imaging and upper endoscopy, as well as a nuclear medicine gastric emptying study in which a patient ingests radiolabeled food and emptying time is documented.

Constipation is a commonly encountered cause of abdominal pain. Patients may note infrequent bowel movements but may also note daily bowel movements that are small and leave them with a sense of incomplete evacuation. If constipation is suspected, abdominal X-ray can be done to assess stool burden.

Elevated Liver Function Tests

Many rheumatologic medications require monitoring of liver tests. Elevation of the aminotransferases suggests hepatocellular injury, while elevation of the alkaline phosphate suggests a biliary pathology. For mild to moderate elevation of aminotransferases, initial evaluation should include testing for hepatitis B and C, iron, and iron saturation to test for hemochromatosis and imaging, such as RUQ ultrasound, to evaluate for steatosis, or fat, in the liver. If these evaluations are negative, testing for autoimmune hepatitis, Wilson disease, alpha-1 anti-trypsin disease, thyroid disease, and celiac disease may be indicated. For those patients with elevated alkaline phosphatase, evaluation should first include confirmation that the elevation of alkaline phosphatase is of liver origin, which can be done through ordering a fractionated alkaline phosphatase to determine the proportion of bone- and liver-related enzyme, and a GGT (gamma glutamyl transpeptidase), which is found in hepatocytes and biliary cells. If elevated alkaline phosphatase is thought to be of liver origin, initial evaluation should include an RUQ ultrasound to evaluate the biliary system.

CONCLUSION

Patients often report gastrointestinal symptoms to their rheumatologist. Consideration can be given to testing for infectious causes of acute diarrhea, particularly when immunosuppression is present. If a high index of suspicion for inflammatory diarrhea exists, sending a fecal calprotectin and taking a careful history may be good starting points in evaluation. Dysphagia usually requires GI referral for endoscopic evaluation, followed by manometry if negative. SIBO may be encountered in patients with slowed GI motility and can be tested for with glucose or lactose breath tests, or in cases where motility is a known factor, it is reasonable to empirically treat. Abdominal pain is common in the population, and initial consideration for *H. pylori* testing, followed by treatment with acid suppression therapy or management of constipation, is reasonable if no alarm symptoms are present. Liver tests are often followed in clinical practice, and Rheumatologists frequently detect abnormalities. If these do not reverse with medication cessation, some initial testing may be done before hepatology referral, such as testing for hepatitis B and C, which immunosuppressive therapy may reactivate, and imaging of the liver with RUQ ultrasound.

REFERENCES

1. Sperber AD, Bangdiwala SI, Drossman DA et al. Worldwide prevalence and burden of functional gastrointestinal disorders, results of Rome Foundation Global Study. *Gastroenterol.* 2021;160(1):99–114. PMID: 32294476
2. Waugh N, Cummins E, Royle P et al. Faecal calprotectin for differentiating amongst inflammatory and non inflammatory bowel diseases: Systematic review and economic evaluation. *Health Technol Assess.* 2013 Nov;17(55):xv–xix, 1–211. PMC4781415
3. Vanga R, Tansel A, Sidiq S et al. Diagnostic performance of measurement of fecal elastase-1 in detection of exocrine pancreatic insufficiency: Systematic review and meta-analysis. *Clin Gastroenterol Hepatol.* 2018 Aug;16(8):1220–8.e4. PMC6402774
4. Robb B, Matthews J. Bile salt diarrhea. *Curr Gastorenterol Rep.* 2005;7(5):379–83. PMID: 16168236
5. Pimentel M, Saad R, Long M et al. ACG clinical guideline: Small intestinal bacterial overgrowth. *Am J Gastroenterol.* 2020;115(2):165–78. PMID: 32023228
6. Talley N, Ford A. Functional dyspepsia. *N Engl J Med.* 2015;373(19):1853–63. PMID: 26535514

2

Fundamental Principles of Gastrointestinal Imaging and Testing

ADAM C. STEIN

INTRODUCTION

While paramount to health and wellness, the gastrointestinal (GI) system is also one of the most commonly impacted areas of the body by diseases and disorders, accounting for a significant proportion of healthcare-related expenses arising in both the acute-care and outpatient settings (1). Efficient evaluation and management of the GI system is essential to providing a timely diagnosis, evidence-based effective treatment, and managing associated costs.

Evaluation of the GI system is typically a linear process based on the combination of descriptive signs and symptoms as well as available objective data. Key to this evaluation is gathering relevant clinical information from a focused yet thorough history and physical examination, which will guide development of a focused differential and dictate subsequent testing as indicated (2). In obtaining a history, one should focus on the timing of symptom onset as well as potential related events. For example, when evaluating someone for diarrhea, it is important to understand the onset of diarrhea and the characteristics of the diarrhea as well as determining surrounding factors including if there has been exposure to others with similar symptoms, travel, or any possible foodborne exposure. Physical examination should include evaluation of the abdomen as well as any other associated symptoms that could provide relevant data; evaluating for "extraintestinal" manifestations of suspected

inflammatory bowel disease should include skin, joint, eye, and mouth exams. A detailed review of history and physical exam components as well as formulating a differential diagnosis is detailed in other parts of this book. This chapter will focus on various testing strategies to gather data in an effort to help understand the diagnosis and evolution of the patient's presenting illness as well as potential therapeutic benefits embedded in some of the tests that one can employ for gastrointestinal illnesses. This consists of three principal areas: laboratory analysis, imaging, and procedures.

LABORATORY ANALYSIS

After a focused history and physical examination, laboratory analysis can provide helpful data to either help guide further testing or secure a diagnosis. Routine laboratory testing for GI disorders typically involves blood/serum or stool-based analysis. Determining which labs to order is based on the history of present illness and, as such, is presented in this manner.

Blood/Serum Testing

Complete Blood Count (CBC) measures several components of circulating blood cells, including white blood cells (WBC), markers of blood oxygen delivery (hemoglobin, hematocrit), and platelets.

White Blood Cells (WBC) An abnormal WBC could indicate infection or inflammation, or indicate

DOI: 10.1201/9781003367307-2

medication use such as steroids. Further breakdown of the total WBC into different types of cells such as neutrophils, lymphocytes, and eosinophils can help hone a differential. For example, an elevated eosinophil count could indicate a parasitic-type infection or could indicate an inflammatory disorder characterized by an eosinophil-predominant cell pattern at the tissue level such as eosinophilic enteritis (3, 4). Medication use should be taken into account when interpreting WBC, as steroids or immunomodulators can cause an abnormal WBC value. Notably, infections or inflammatory conditions may not cause an abnormal WBC and/or cell type differential, and as such, the WBC and differential should not be interpreted in isolation.

Hemoglobin/Hematocrit and other markers evaluating the size, shape, and maturity of red blood cells (RBCs) are necessary to diagnose anemia and other blood-related disorders that the GI system can potentially impact. Anemia is a common cause of morbidity associated with the GI system through either intestinal bleeding or malabsorption of components required to produce mature RBCs. While a deep dive into the components of red blood cells measured in a CBC is outside the scope of this practice, typically, a low hemoglobin/hematocrit is further delineated based on the size and shape of circulating red blood cells (macrocytic, normocytic, and microcytic). A normocytic anemia could be due to acute blood loss. A macrocytic anemia could indicate malabsorption of vitamin B12 or folate, leading to decreased RBC production. A microcytic anemia is indicative of low iron levels and/or chronic blood loss. In the setting of acute bleeding, such as seen with the GI system, one may potentially find the hemoglobin/hematocrit level is within a normal range due to whole blood being lost; repeat analysis after some time has passed will allow for equilibration and a more accurate value, which may reveal anemia.

Platelets are an essential part of the clotting cascade, an important measurement when evaluating the GI system. Low platelets may indicate decreased ability to form a clot and thus may cause delays in procedures due to procedure-related bleeding risk if platelets are below a critical threshold (5). High platelets may be an indirect indicator of an inflammatory state (6).

Basic Metabolic Panel (BMP) is a measurement of kidney function (blood urea nitrogen (BUN) and creatinine), basic electrolytes (sodium, potassium), buffer of acid/base status (bicarbonate), and glucose. From a GI standpoint, the BMP is helpful in a few scenarios. For GI bleeding, an elevated BUN that is out of proportion to creatinine could indicate a source proximal to the ligament of Trietz (upper GI bleeding) (7). Kidney function can be helpful with dosing and monitoring renally excreted medications.

Liver Tests, often referred to as 'liver function tests' (LFTs), measure markers of the hepatic parenchyma (alanine transaminase [ALT] and aspartate transaminase [AST]), synthetic function (albumin), and the hepatobiliary system (total bilirubin, alkaline phosphatase (sometimes referred to as 'alk phos' or ALP). Elevated ALT and/or AST can be seen in acute and chronic liver disease including hepatitis. The ratio of AST to ALT can be useful in determining if there is a component of alcoholic steatohepatitis versus nonalcoholic steatohepatitis (or fatty liver disease) (8). An abnormally elevated total bilirubin is rather ambiguous from a diagnostic standpoint, and understanding the production can help hone the differential. Bilirubin is predominately sourced from the breakdown of red blood cells; it is then taken up by hepatocytes, then modified ('conjugated'), and finally secreted into bile that is then delivered to the small intestine via the hepatobiliary system. Measuring the conjugated (direct) or unconjugated (indirect) versions of bilirubin can help determine the source of elevation (9). A predominately unconjugated elevation indicates increased rate of hemolysis, or malfunctioning hepatocytes. Direct bilirubin elevation indicates an issue after conjugation in the hepatocytes, typically in the hepatobiliary excretion (including biliary blockage) (9). Alkaline phosphatase is another lab with significant nuance; many tissues make ALP, including the liver, bone, intestines, and kidneys (10). Alkaline phosphatase can be analyzed for these metabolites, or isoenzymes. From a GI standpoint, an elevated liver-specific ALP isoenzyme can indicate damage to the hepatobiliary system, especially if there is an associated increase in bilirubin.

Inflammatory Markers. There are several measurable markers of inflammation; most are non-specific and have variable sensitivities and specificities. Testing includes direct measurements of inflammation, c-reactive protein (CRP), and erythrocyte sedimentation rate (ESR), as well as indirect measurements of inflammation in the form of 'acute phase reactant' markers. Acute phase reactants are lab values that either increase or decrease in the setting of systemic inflammation. Examples include vitamin D, platelets, albumin (11–13). Both CRP and ESR are commonly measured when intestinal inflammation is suspected or to follow the trajectory and severity of established inflammation (13).

Infectious Diseases. There is significant burden of infectious diseases impacting the GI system throughout the world, manifesting most commonly as either upper GI symptoms (nausea/vomiting, abdominal discomfort) or diarrhea (which can also include abdominal discomfort) (14). Specifics of when to test and what organisms to test for are outside the scope of this chapter. If testing is indicated, there are several different types of tests for stool pathogens available, all of which are stool-based tests (blood-/serum-based testing can be used as evidence of systemic spread, as in CMV, or confirmation of prior exposure, as in *Helicobacter pylori*). Tests available are dependent on location and resources. Tests historically have assessed a single or a cluster of infectious organisms; newer available tests are more comprehensive in nature, testing for many infections using one sample.

Stool Analysis (Diarrhea). Evaluation of diarrhea is typically broken down into three time periods: acute (diarrhea for less than 2 weeks), persistent (diarrhea for 2 to 4 weeks), and chronic (diarrhea present for at least 4 weeks) (15). Alternatively, diarrhea can be quantified by fecal volume of at least 200 ml or weight over 200 g in a 24-hour period (16). Testing for acute diarrhea, when indicated, is typically to evaluate for infectious organisms. When diarrhea progresses beyond acute, testing may broaden beyond infectious etiologies. Assessing for noninfectious diarrhea is often non-specific in terms of exact etiology but can help provide data to focus further evaluation. There are three different types of analytic categories that can be performed on stool beyond infection: osmolality (osmotic/secretory), inflammation, and malabsorption.

Osmolality. The causes of diarrhea can be further divided into three types based on electrolyte measurements in the stool compared to serum osmolality: secretory, osmotic, or mixed. To gain accuracy, electrolytes are typically measured on stool collected over a period of time (usually 24 to 72 hours) to avoid misleading results. Sodium (Na^+) and potassium (K^-) are necessary to measure for osmolality, while magnesium (Mg^{2+}) can also be measured to assess for laxative use containing Mg^{2+}. Stool osmolality is calculated by taking the serum osmolality (either measured or using the estimation of 290 mOsm/L) and subtracting the doubled product of adding stool Na^+ and K- ($290 - 2x(Na^+ + K^-)$). A result below 50 indicates a secretory process, and above 50 indicates either an osmotic or mixed secretory/osmotic process.

Inflammation. Detecting inflammatory markers in the stool is helpful in establishing the presence of inflammation. However, these tests are generally regarded as non-specific for etiology and are limited by relatively low sensitivity and specificity, leading to potential falsely negative results. The two mainstays for fecal inflammatory markers are direct visualization of white blood cells (WBC, or leukocytes) and indirect presence via assay of the neutrophil-specific marker calprotectin (17–19). Both of these markers can help determine if inflammation is present in the GI system, but neither is specific for any one cause, and they can be positive in the setting of overt bleeding (19).

Malabsorption. Diarrhea caused by malabsorption of a particular compound, typically either fat, protein, carbohydrate, or other ingested product, can be performed by stool-based analysis. Steatorrhea (fat malabsorption) can be assessed by direct visualization and quantification of fat in stool. Spot testing via direct visualization can establish the presence of fat in stool. However, there can be small amounts of fat in healthy stool. As such, visualization is typically not enough to establish fat malabsorption. Additionally, lack of fat in the diet can also lead to falsely negative results. As such, testing is done via a 24- to 72-hour stool collection and on a high-fat diet to avoid false negative results. Normal stool can have up to 7 grams of fat over a 24-hour period. More than 7 g indicates likely fat malabsorption. One etiology of fat malabsorption is pancreatic exocrine insufficiency. This can be established by measuring a stool-based enzyme called fecal elastase. The presence of fecal elastase in abundance is normal (usually reported as above 200 μg/g), whereas a lower value of elastase in the stool can indicate pancreatic exocrine insufficiency. As with other stool testing for diarrhea, fasting or a modified diet (in this case, a low-fat diet) can cause false positive results due to the pancreas not needing to secrete a normal level of enzymes. Protein is typically not a cause of malabsorption, but it can be excreted in the setting of inflammation (enteropathy). Stool-based testing can be done for this via an alpha-1-antitrypsin clearance. This test involves measuring stool alpha-1-antitrypsin over a 24-hour period and comparing to the serum level of alpha-1-antitrypsin during the same time period. The calculation for this is stool volume in grams multiplied by the stool alpha-1-antitrypsin value (both over 24 hours), then divided by the serum alpha-1-antitrypsin level. Normal clearance is defined as less than 13 mL/day. False results can be seen in the setting of liver disease or genetic variants, as alpha-1-antitrypsin is produced in the liver and is prone to genetic variants that decrease production. Carbohydrate malabsorption is assessed by breath-based testing using the carbohydrate in question (lactose, fructose, sucrose).

Vitamin/Mineral testing can be used to assess for deficiencies or toxicities. Within GI, several are implicated in different disease processes.

Vitamin A can be low in the setting of fat malabsorption or malnutrition, and toxicity is typically seen with ingestion of excess vitamin A, usually in a medication or supplement form. There are multiple metabolites of vitamin A in the body and also tissue; typically, testing is done on one metabolite called retinol. Given so many metabolites and storage in tissue, testing is not necessarily accurate (20). Testing is serum based.

Vitamin B12 deficiency can be seen in a variety of GI disorders and can lead to anemia. It is absorbed in a two-step process. First, vitamin B12 is bound to a protein called intrinsic factor, which is produced in the stomach. The complex is then absorbed into the body in the terminal ileum. An abnormality in either the stomach or distal small bowel can impact absorption and thus lead to vitamin B12 deficiency. Laboratory clues for vitamin B12 deficiency include a high MCV level (macrocytosis). Testing is serum based.

Folate is another cause of an elevated MCV and anemia when deficient. Testing is serum based.

Vitamin D deficiency is linked to inflammation in the bowel, specifically inflammatory bowel disease (21). Vitamin D is also a reverse acute phase reactant, meaning the measured level can decrease in the setting of inflammation (22). Vitamin D has several metabolites in the body (23). Typically, one of the precursor metabolites is measured in serum,

25-hydroxyvitamin D. The metabolically active compound 1,25-dihydroxyvitamin D can also be measured in patients suspected to have decreased metabolism of vitamin D, typically in patients with kidney disease.

Iron deficiency is a common referral to gastroenterologists, as iron is absorbed in the proximal small bowel and can be lost due to inflammation or bleeding within the GI tract. Laboratory clues for iron deficiency typically include anemia and/or a low MCV level. There are several tests that can assess iron deficiency, including total serum iron level, ferritin, and total iron binding capacity (TIBC). Of note, ferritin is an acute phase reactant and can rise in the setting of inflammation; caution should be taken in interpreting a ferritin level in the setting of systemic inflammation, as a normal-range ferritin may actually be falsely normal (24).

IMAGING

Imaging the abdomen is often a useful tool in helping to determine the cause of a person's gastrointestinal signs/symptoms. Imaging can take the form of traditional two-dimensional views (X-ray, ultrasound) or three-dimensional (CT, MRI, PET) studies. Dynamic imaging that evaluates the flow of ingested contrast over time can also be performed via fluoroscopic two-dimensional imaging (esophogram/SBFT). While most imaging tests are relatively quick and innocuous, there may be potential harm from radiation exposure and intravenous contrast use (25–26).

X-Ray

A static two-dimensional image of the abdomen and/or pelvis can be done via X-ray. This test is typically done without any ingested contrast and can be done with the patient in various positions to allow for visualization of changes to the air and fluid within the GI system. This quick, noninvasive test is often the initial study when a patient presents with a question of bowel obstruction or bowel perforation.

Fluoroscopy

A real-time imaging study using two-dimensional X-ray called fluoroscopy can be done to evaluate the anatomic and luminal structures of the GI tract. Common studies include esophogram (evaluation of contrast movement through the mouth and esophagus), upper GI series (esophogram plus evaluation of the stomach), small bowel follow-through (assessment of contrast through the small bowel), and barium enema (evaluation of the colon).

Ultrasound

Ultrasound images are generated by sound waves penetrating and deflecting off tissue in the body. From a GI perspective, ultrasound has traditionally been utilized to evaluate the pancreaticobiliary system and liver, with recent advances showing promise in evaluating the intestinal system as well. Blood flow can also be evaluated via doppler ultrasonography. Ultrasound can also be performed luminally, as done with an endoscope (endoscopic ultrasound), which is discussed in more detail elsewhere in this chapter.

With direct visualization, the gallbladder, biliary ducts, pancreas, and pancreatic ducts can all be seen in good detail. Ultrasound is useful for identifying anatomical issues, stones, lesions, or inflammation. The limitations of ultrasound for these areas include decreased visualization from overlying bowel or other anatomical abnormalities including altered anatomy from surgery.

Liver ultrasound can screen for liver lesions such as abscesses, cysts, or malignancies. Liver ultrasound can also evaluate the texture (echogenicity) of the liver parenchyma, assessing for fat infiltration (fatty liver) or scar tissue (cirrhosis). Typically, ultrasound of the liver provides evidence of underlying pathology, but it is not usually considered enough to provide a diagnosis; other testing is usually required to confirm any visualized abnormality.

Computed Tomography (CT)

Cross-sectional imaging of the abdomen and pelvis can be performed via a series of X-rays that are computer processed to generate a three-dimensional view of the body in the form of computer tomography (CT). There are multiple ways to "protocol" the CT to view the GI system, with and without contrast (oral and/or intravenous [IV]). A standard CT of the abdomen and pelvis uses iodinated IV contrast and ingested (oral) contrast with a base of either iodine or barium. The scanner will then take various images during different time points based on both oral ingestion and injection via IV to enhance certain features of the GI tract. Features that can be enhanced using this protocol are anatomical structures of the GI tract as well as the vascular system in the abdomen/pelvis (27). A CT scan is useful to get an outline of the GI system to assess potential anatomical issues such as blockages or mass lesions or to provide finer detail of the vascular system for bleeding, ischemia, or vascular-type lesions such as polyps or masses. Changing the iodinated or barium oral contrast to lower density or even contrast-neutral water-based solution provides finer detail of the enteric mucosa. This protocol (CT enterography) typically allows for a more detailed view of bowel mucosa, assessing for evidence of luminal inflammation in processes such as Crohn's disease (28).

Magnetic Resonance Imaging (MRI)

Another modality to evaluate the GI system involves using computer-generated radio waves within a magnetic field to produce an image based on movement of protons in the body during magnetic exposure. No radiation is involved in producing the images. However, gadolinium-based IV contrast can be used to aid in image generation. Different types of oral contrast can be used to enhance the bowel, including enterography protocol similar to CT scans.

Positron Emission Tomography (PET)

Positron emission tomography (PET), often combined with CT (PET/CT), provides another modality to assess the GI system free from radiation. Fundamentally, PET scanning involves using a radiotracer to quantify metabolic activity, providing a map based on changes in glucose metabolism (29). Different radiotracers can be used, including the glucose metabolism marker fluorodeoxyglucose (FDG), and gallium-68 DOTATATE (dotatate), which is utilized for somatostatin metabolism (29–30). Both radiotracers are able to detect increased metabolic activity in the GI system, with FDG acting in a relatively nonspecific variety, and they can assess for malignancy as well as inflammation. Dotatate is quite specific for neuroendocrine tumors (30–32). Currently, PET is only recommended for evaluation of malignancy. However, utilization as a tool for GI inflammatory conditions may be reasonable based on accumulating evidence (32).

Nuclear

Imaging of the GI system can also be accomplished using harmless radioactive materials, either consumed orally (or through an enteral tube) or intravenously. There are several nuclear tests:

Gastric Emptying Scan involves eating or drinking a radiolabeled meal and evaluating how quickly the radiolabeled contents empty out of the stomach. This is typically presented as percent cleared and is done over a several-hour period of time.

Tagged Red Blood Cell Scan (also called a bleeding scan) evaluates potential GI bleeding by marking red blood cells with a radiotracer and seeing if the radiotracer enters the GI lumen. This test can be done over a several-hour period. A positive test requires active bleeding at a brisk enough rate so that the scanning system can pick up luminal flow.

Meckel's Scan evaluates for a Meckel's diverticula, which is a congenital diverticula located in the distal small bowel, typically containing ectopic gastric mucosa, and can cause bleeding or inflammation of the distal small bowel or colon. The scan involves using an intravenous radiotracer that preferentially is taken up by gastric tissue. While the sensitivity of a positive Meckel's scan nears 100%, the specificity decreases with age, and has been reported to be lower than 50% in adults (33).

Hepatobiliary Iminodiacetic Acid (HIDA) Scan evaluates for biliary pathology, specifically a blockage in bile flow from the liver to the small bowel. This involves using a radiotracer that is taken up by hepatocytes and secreted into bile. An abnormal test can be seen in a variety of pathology involving the hepatobiliary system, including cholecystitis, biliary obstruction, or congenital bile duct disorders such as biliary atresia.

ENDOSCOPY

Direct visualization of the GI system as well as the partial visualization of the biliary system can be accomplished by endoscopic assessment. Endoscopy accomplishes two main things: direct evaluation of anatomy and mucosa lining the GI tract for diagnostic purposes and therapeutic interventions employed directly via endoscopic techniques. Typically, endoscopic evaluation involves sedation for patient comfort. However, many techniques can also be performed without sedation if needed or by patient preference. Sedation can be done by the endoscopist or by an anesthesiology team. Risks of endoscopy are determined by the procedure as well as any diagnostic or therapeutic maneuvers. Common risks include bleeding and perforation; risks are quite rare and are mitigated by operator experience as well as medication management. Further device-specific risks are noted in what follows. Detailed uses of these different endoscopic techniques are included in other chapters.

Esophagogastroduodenoscopy (EGD)

Evaluation of the esophagus, stomach, and proximal portion of the small intestine (typically limited to the duodenum or proximal jejunum, as is the case with a "push" enteroscopy) is accomplished by EGD. This allows for direct visualization of potential pathology as well as a variety of diagnostic and therapeutic maneuvers. Tissue can be sampled via forceps for biopsy or brushing for cells. Emerging techniques allow for more direct cellular visualization via different types of light filters as well as instruments that can be deployed directly onto tissue (34–35). From a therapeutic standpoint, there are multiple instruments and techniques available to remove tissue including polyps, injecting medication, dilating strictures, and stopping or preventing bleeding.

Flexible Sigmoidoscopy/Colonoscopy

As with EGD, visualization of the colon and distal small bowel (terminal ileum) is accomplished using colonoscopy. Flexible sigmoidoscopy is a variety of colonoscopy, where the operator limits endoscopic assessment to the colon distal to the splenic flexure. Both colonoscopy and flexible sigmoidoscopy are used for both diagnostic and therapeutic purposes, as detailed earlier in the EGD section.

Enteroscopy

Visualizing the entirety of the small bowel was traditionally accomplished by intraoperative enteroscopy, where the endoscope was passed directly through the small bowel through a purposeful enterotomy during abdominal surgery. This technique has now been replaced by device-assisted enteroscopy (DAE). DAE allows for direct endoscopic visualization of the deeper portions of small bowel not typically reached by standard EGD or colonoscopy, entering the GI tract through the mouth, stoma, or anus. There are two main techniques to accomplish this: balloon-assisted or spiral technique. Both techniques are diagnostic as well as therapeutic in nature, including what can be done via EGD or colonoscopy. Both techniques are considered safe and effective, but require specialized training and/or operator experience, and are typically available only at specialized endoscopy centers.

Video Capsule Endoscopy (VCE)

Also known as wireless capsule endoscopy (WCE), this non-absorbed pill with at least one camera is swallowed (or placed endoscopically) and takes thousands of pictures as it tumbles through the GI system. These images are either wirelessly transmitted to a receiver in real time or transmitted to a computer after capsule retrieval once passed via stool. Three different types of VCEs are available (esophagus, small bowel, and colon) and are used to assess the lumen and mucosa of the targeted GI area of choice. Video capsule endoscopy can be used in combination with or in lieu of standard endoscopic techniques (EGD, colonoscopy, enteroscopy). The most common use of VCE is for small bowel evaluation prior to enteroscopy, typically in the setting of suspected small bowel bleeding (36). Other common reasons for small bowel VCE include inflammatory evaluation as well as assessment for premalignant or malignant changes. Esophageal and colonic visualization are not commonly performed but are also available.

Three important considerations exist for VCE. First, the operator has no control of how the VCE passes through the GI system and also no ability to perform therapeutic maneuvers, although emerging technology may allow for more direct control of the capsule in the future. This lack of control leads to risk of missing pathology, as the camera (or cameras) may not capture a clear or direct image of any abnormalities. As such, the sensitivity and specificity of VCE does not reach 100% and is often quoted (depending on the type of pathology) to be significantly less (37–38). Secondly, the VCE is housed in a nondissolvable casing. This may lead to VCE retention, necessitating capsule retrieval by either endoscopy or surgery. History of abdominal surgery, prior abdominal radiation, or bowel obstruction should all give pause to the provider due to increased risk of capsule retention, and further investigation should be undertaken prior to any VCE exam. A variety of different methods are available to determine the risk associated with VCE retention. Recent small bowel imaging with good luminal expansion with oral contrast showing no evidence of obstruction or narrowing is associated with low risk of capsule retention (39–40). A dissolvable patency capsule can also be used to assess passage; the patency capsule is swallowed, then 1 to 2 days later, an imaging study is performed to see where the capsule is located. If the capsule is located in the colon or is found to have passed through the entire GI system, the likelihood of capsule retention is also lowered. Anecdotally, VCE retention may be somewhat diagnostic in nature, as retention may be at a site of pathology. Third, VCE is contraindicated in the setting of implanted cardiac devices including pacemakers and defibrillators. This is in part due to potential interference with the cardiac device while the VCE wirelessly transmits images. To this date, there is a paucity of reported interference with VCEs and implanted cardiac devices (41–42). As such, many gastroenterologists are comfortable with doing VCE in this setting, using a variety of different protocols to mitigate risk. Detailed assessment of these protocols is beyond the scope of this chapter.

Endoscopic Ultrasound (EUS)

Luminal ultrasound of the GI and hepatobiliary systems can be accomplished using a specialized endoscope with an ultrasound probe, available for both EGD and colonoscopy. Luminal ultrasound allows for inspection of the submucosal tissue not normally visualized during endoscopic assessment. Many indications exist for EUS and are detailed in other chapters. Like enteroscopy, EUS is typically only available at specialized endoscopic centers.

Endoscopic Retrograde Cholangiopancreatography (ERCP)

The hepatobiliary system can be further evaluated by ERCP, which involves direct cannulation of the common bile duct and/or pancreatic ducts via the ampulla in the duodenum. Once cannulated, instruments can be deployed to visualize the ducts using fluoroscopy. Both diagnostic and therapeutic options are available during ERCP, including brushing, biopsy, sweeping the duct, and deploying stents to open a narrowed duct or prevent further narrowing from occurring. Risks of ERCP include bleeding, infection, biliary perforation, and pancreatitis (43).

CONCLUSION

A plethora of tools are available to evaluate the GI system. Which modalities to use typically evolves after first performing a focused history and physical examination. Options range from noninvasive laboratory assessments and imaging studies to more invasive endoscopic examinations. All have the potential to help with diagnosis, while some have the ability to provide therapy as well.

REFERENCES

1. Peery AF, Crockett SD, Murphy CC et al. Burden and cost of gastrointestinal, liver, and pancreatic diseases in the United States: Update 2018. *Gastroenterol.* 2019 Jan;156(1):254–72. PMC6689327

2. Wang TC, Camilleri M, Lebwohl B et al. *Yamada's textbook of gastroenterology.* 1st ed. Hoboken, NJ: John Wiley & Sons Ltd.; 2022.

3. Khanna V, Tilak K, Mukhopadhyay C et al. Significance of diagnosing parasitic infestation in evaluation of unexplained eosinophilia. *J Clin Diagn Res.* 2015 Jul; 9(7):DC22–24. PMC4572961.

4. Dellon ES, Gonsalves N, Abonia JP et al. International consensus recommendations for eosinophilic gastrointestinal disease nomenclature. *Clin Gastroenterol Hepatol.* 2022 Nov;20(11):2474–84. PMC9378753

5. Ross WA. Endoscopic interventions in patients with thrombocytopenia. *Gastroenterol Hepatol (NY).* 2015 Feb;11(2):115–7. PMC4836569

6. Stokes KY, Granger DN. Platelets: A critical link between inflammation and microvascular dysfunction. *J Physiol.* 2012 Mar 1;590(5):1023–34. PMC3381810

7. Ziabari SMZ, Rimaz S, Shafaghi A et al. Blood urea nitrogen to creatinine ratio in differentiation of upper and lower gastrointestinal bleedings; a diagnostic accuracy study. *Arch Acad Emerg Med.* 2019 Jun 2;7(1):e30. PMC6637801

8. Hall P, Cash J. What is the real function of the liver 'function' tests. *Ulster Med J.* 2012 Jan;81(1):30–6. PMC3609680

9. Van Wagner LB, Green RM. Evaluating elevated bilirubin levels in asymptomatic adults. *JAMA.* 2015 Feb 3;313(5):516–7. PMC4424929

10. Crofton PM. Biochemistry of alkaline phosphatase isoenzymes. *Crit Rev Clin Lab Sci.* 1982;16(3):161–94. PMID: 7047076

11. Kasperska-Zajac A, Grzanka A, Jarzab J et al. The association between platelet count and acute phase response in chronic spontaneous urticaria. *Biomed Res Int.* 2014:2014:650913. PMC4084584

12. Gulhar R, Ashraf MA, Jialal I. *StatPearls [Internet].* St. Petersburg, FL: StatPearls Publishing; 2023.

13. Vermeire S, Van Assche G, Rutgeerts P. Laboratory markers in IBD: Useful, magic, or unnecessary toys? *Gut.* 2006 Mar;55(3):426–31. PMC1856093

14. Hatchette TF, Farina D. Infectious diarrhea: When to test and when to treat. *CMAJ.* 2011 Feb 22;183(3):339–44. PMC3042443

15. World Health Organization. 2017. www.who.int/news-room/fact-sheets/detail/diarrhoeal-disease

16. Sweetser S. Evaluating the patient with diarrhea: A case-based approach. *Mayo Clin Proc.* 2012 Jun;87(6):596–602. PMC353847

17. van Rheenen PF, Van de Vijver E, Fidler V. Faecal calprotectin for screening of patients with suspected inflammatory bowel disease: Diagnostic meta-analysis. *BMJ.* 2010 Jul 15;341:c3369. PMC29048

18. Lehmann FS, Burri E, Beglinger C. The role and utility of faecal markers in inflammatory bowel disease. *Therap Adv Gastroenterol.* 2015 Jan;8(1):23–36. PMC4265086

19. Pathirana WGW, Chubb SP, Gillet MJ et al. Faecal calprotectin. *Clin Biochem Rev.* 2018 Aug;39(3):77–90. PMC6370282

20. Greaves RF, Woollard GA, Hoad KE et al. Laboratory medicine best practice guideline: Vitamins A, E and the carotenoids in blood. *Clin Biochem Rev.* 2014 May;35(2):81–113. PMC4159783

21. Fletcher J, Cooper SC, Ghosh S et al. The role of vitamin D in inflammatory bowel disease: Mechanism to management. *Nutrients.* 2019 May 7;11(5):1019. PMC6566188

22. Waldron JL, Ashby HL, Cornes MP et al. Vitamin D: A negative acute phase reactant. *J Clin Pathol.* 2013 Jul; 66(7):620–2. PMID: 23454726

23. Bikle DD. Vitamin D metabolism, mechanism of action, and clinical applications. *Chem Biol.* 2014 20;21(3):319–29. PMC3968073

24. Wang W, Knovich MA, Coffman LG et al. Serum ferritin: Past, present and future. *Biochim Biophys Acta.* 2010 Aug;1800(8):760–9. PMC2893236

25. Nguyen PK, Wu JC. Radiation exposure from imaging tests: Is there an increased cancer risk? *Expert Rev Cardiovasc Ther.* 2011 Feb;9(2):177–83. PMC3102578

26. Baerlocher MO, Asch M, Myers A. The use of contrast media. *CMAJ.* 2010 Apr 20;182(7):697. PMC2934800

27. Pickhardt PJ. Positive oral contrast material for abdominal CT: Current clinical indications and areas of controversy. *AJR Am J Roentgenol.* 2020 Jul;215(1):69–78. PMID: 31913069

28. Ilangovan R, Burling D, George A et al. CT enterography: Review of technique and practical tips. *Br J Radiol.* 2012 Jul; 85(1015):876–86. PMC3474054

29. van Kouwen MCA, Oyen WJG, Nagengast FM et al. FDG-PET scanning in the diagnosis of gastrointestinal cancers. *Scand J Gastroenterol Supp.* 2004:39(241):85–92. PMID: 15696855

30. Raj N, Reidy-Lagunes D. The role of 68Ga-DOTATATE positron emission tomography/computed tomography in well-differentiated neuroendocrine tumors: A case-based approach illustrates potential benefits and challenges. *Pancreas.* 2018 Jan;47(1):1–5. PMC5729934

31. Menon N, Mandelkern M. Utility of PET scans in the diagnosis and management of gastrointestinal tumors. *Dig Dis Sci.* 2022 Oct;67(10):4633–53. PMID: 35908126

32. Brodersen JB, Hess S. FDG-PET/CT in inflammatory bowel disease: Is there a future? *PET Clin.* 2020 Apr;15(2):153–62. PMID: 32145886

33. Hong SN, Jang HJ, Ye BD et al. Diagnosis of bleeding Meckel's diverticulum in adults. *PLoS One.* 2016 Sep 14;11(9):e0162615. PMC5023169

34. Hajelssedig OE, Pu LZCT, Thompson JY et al. Diagnostic accuracy of narrow-band imaging endoscopy with targeted biopsies compared with standard endoscopy with random biopsies in patients with Barrett's esophagus: A systematic review and meta-analysis. *J Gastroenterol Hepatol.* 2021 Oct; 36(10):2659–71. PMID: 34121232

35. Chauhan SS, Dayyeh BKA, Bhat YM et al. Confocal laser endomicroscopy. *Gastrointest Endosc.* 2014 Dec;80(6):928–38. PMID: 25442092

36. Gerson LB, Fidler JL, Cave DR et al. ACG clinical guideline: Diagnosis and management of small bowel bleeding. *Am J Gastroenterol.* 2015 Sep;110(9):1265–87. PMID: 26303132

37. Cheung DY, Kim JS, Shim KN et al. The usefulness of capsule endoscopy for small bowel tumor. *Clin Endosc.* 2016 Jan;49(1):21–5. PMID: 26855919

38. Pasha SF, Leighton JA. Evidence-based guide on capsule endoscopy for small bowel bleeding. *Gastroenterol Hepatol (NY).* 2017 Feb;13(2):88–93. PMC5402689

39. Rondonotti E. Capsule retention: Prevention, diagnosis and management. *Ann Transl Med.* 2017 May;5(9):198. PMID: 28567378

40. Rezapour M, Amadi C, Gerson LB. Retention associated with video capsule endoscopy: Systematic review and meta-analysis. *Gastrointest Endosc.* 2017 Jun;85(6):1157–68. PMID: 28069475

41. Tabet R, Nassani N, Karam B et al. Pooled analysis of the efficacy and safety of video capsule endoscopy in patients

with implantable cardiac devices. *Can J Gastroenterol Hepatol*. 2019 May 19:2019:3953807. PMID: 31236386

42. Leighton JA, Sharma VK, Srivathsan K et al. Safety of capsule endoscopy in patients with pacemakers. *Gastrointest Endosc*. 2004 Apr;59(4):567–9. PMID: 15044901

43. Szary NM, Al-Kawas FH. Complications of endoscopic retrograde cholangiopan-creatography: How to avoid and manage them. *Gastroenterol Hepatol* (NY). 2013 Aug;9(8):496–504. PMC3980992

3

Rheumatoid Arthritis and Sjogren's Disease

MICHAEL CAMMARATA AND REEM JAN

RHEUMATOID ARTHRITIS

Introduction

Rheumatoid arthritis is chronic inflammatory joint disease that is characterized by synovial proliferation and erosive cartilage and joint destruction. The prevalence in the US is around 0.5%, with a female preponderance. Diagnosis is based on a history of painful swollen joints and prolonged morning stiffness, physical findings of synovitis, and laboratory testing that shows elevated rheumatoid factor and anti-CCP antibodies. Seronegative rheumatoid arthritis is well described and may run a more benign clinical course. X-rays of the hands and feet of patients with suspected RA may show uniform joint space narrowing, periarticular osteopenia, and marginal erosions.

The hallmark of rheumatoid arthritis (RA) is synovitis, but it can present with numerous extra-articular features, such as pulmonary, ocular, and cutaneous disease. Gastrointestinal symptoms in patients with rheumatoid arthritis are most often secondary to adverse effects from medications, such as GI upset from DMARDs like methotrexate and ulceration from chronic NSAIDs and high-dose steroids (1). Direct gastrointestinal complications from the disease itself are rare, and seropositive patients with longstanding and often, uncontrolled disease tend to be the most vulnerable group. This section will focus on the gastrointestinal manifestations of three particular entities that can be seen in unchecked rheumatoid arthritis: rheumatoid vasculitis, secondary amyloidosis, and Felty's syndrome with nodular regenerative hyperplasia. We will discuss their incidence and risk factors, pathophysiology, and presentation, as well as diagnosis and treatment.

RHEUMATOID VASCULITIS

Rheumatoid vasculitis (RV) is a heterogenous, predominantly small- and medium-vessel vasculitis that can affect multiple systems including the skin, nerves, eyes, pericardium, lungs, and, rarely, the bowels, kidneys and central nervous system. Rheumatoid vasculitis was first described in the late 19th century with a case of neuritis (2) and later digital gangrene and mononeuritis multiplex (3). Gastrointestinal manifestations of the disease are rare but well documented and extremely varied in presentation. Therefore, clinicians must have a high index of suspicion for the disease in a patient with the appropriate risk factors.

The incidence of rheumatoid vasculitis appears to be declining (4–6). This contrasts with other forms of vasculitis, where the incidence is stable (7). In the longest prospective epidemiological study of rheumatoid vasculitis, the incidence from 2001–2010 was significantly lower than in the previous 1988–2000 cohort (6). This is likely attributable to early and aggressive control of disease activity (8), the use of methotrexate, decreased smoking rates,

DOI: 10.1201/9781003367307-3

and the increase in available therapies with the arrival of the "biologic era" (7).

Risk factors for rheumatoid vasculitis include male sex (5, 9), smoking, and longstanding, seropositive, and erosive disease (6, 10). RV is rare in patients with seronegative RA (11). Longstanding disease is key, considering the mean duration between diagnosis of rheumatoid arthritis and presentation of rheumatoid vasculitis is 10 to 14 years (9, 12). Not all patients will have active synovitis, however, and may present with "burned out" arthritis and low disease activity. Often, they will have co-morbid peripheral arterial disease and cardiovascular disease risk factors (13). Extraarticular manifestations of RA, such as pulmonary fibrosis, share the same risk factors as rheumatoid vasculitis and thus may be seen in patients with RV (7).

Laboratory evaluation for RV is nonspecific and supportive rather than diagnostic. It commonly reveals evidence of chronic inflammation: a normocytic anemia with thrombocytosis, elevated inflammatory markers, and hypocomplementemia, though low complement is not always present (14).

While leukocytoclastic vasculitis, mononeuritis, cutaneous ulceration, nailfold infarcts, and digital gangrene are classic presentations of rheumatoid vasculitis, gastrointestinal manifestations occur on rare occasions and must be kept in mind in the appropriate patient population. The incidence of gastrointestinal disease in RV is estimated at 1% to 10% (15, 16) and likely declining. In the NORVASC cohort, gastrointestinal manifestation represented 10% of cases from 1975–1981, 4% (2/18) of cases from 1988–2000, and 0% from 2001–2010 (6).

Literature detailing the spectrum of GI involvement in RV is limited to case reports and case series. Gastrointestinal manifestations are extremely varied, from mild abdominal pain to life-threatening hemorrhage and peritonitis, but abdominal pain is a common, unifying feature. Given that rheumatoid vasculitis targets the medium vessels of the abdomen, it can mimic polyarteritis nodosa, and the two entities may be difficult to differentiate (17, 18). Presentations of GI disease from RV include ulceration, colitis (19, 20), bowel infarction and necrosis (21, 22), perforation and acute abdomen (23), stricture, and small bowel obstruction (24), as well as ileus (25).

Tago et al. reported a case of a 65-year-old man with a 20-year history of rheumatoid arthritis who presented with recurrent ileal stenosis and small bowel obstruction (SBO) (25). The patient was also noted to have hypocomplementemia. After failure of conservative management of the SBO, the stenotic region of the ileum was surgically removed, and he was found to have multiple mucosal ulcerations due to RV. Kuehne et al. reported a similar case in a 65-year-old man with over 10 years of disease treated with gold, who presented with a SBO due to stricture (24). Rheumatoid vasculitis has been reported as appendicitis (26), as well as hemorrhage, especially when vascular inflammation leads to pseudoaneurysm and rupture. Mizuno et al. reported a case occurring outside of the intestines with intrahepatic hemorrhage due to pseudoaneurysms of the right hepatic artery that were ultimately attributed to vasculitis (27). This patient improved with embolization and corticosteroids. Achkar et al. reported a similar case of a ruptured middle colic artery aneurysm due to RV resulting in hemoperitoneum (28).

Diagnosis of gastrointestinal disease secondary to rheumatoid vasculitis is challenging, especially in the absence of the other cutaneous or peripheral findings characteristic of the disease. Often, a histopathologic diagnosis is made when surgically removed sections of bowel are examined. In the absence of surgical pathology, one must rely on angiography, analogous to PAN, to evaluate for medium-vessel vasculitis. Pseudoaneurysms are inconsistently reported (17, 28), but microaneurysms are not thought to be part of the disease, in contrast with PAN (7). CT imaging may show stricture, colitis, or perforation. Removed tissue should also be stained for amyloid, which can overlap with rheumatoid vasculitis (29) and will be discussed in the following section.

In Pagnoux's analysis of 62 patients presenting with gastrointestinal involvement from systemic necrotizing vasculitides, only three were secondary to rheumatoid vasculitis. All presented with abdominal pain and a surgical abdomen (30). Each of the patients died, highlighting its poor prognosis (15, 16, 31). Despite the decrease in incidence, mortality related to rheumatoid vasculitis has not changed, with 5-year mortality rates around 60% (6, 12).

Management of gastrointestinal related rheumatoid vasculitis is centered around timely surgical management and treatment with high-dose corticosteroids and either rituximab or cyclophosphamide

(9, 32). Given the low incidence, heterogenous presentation, and lack of classification criteria, data on treatment are sparse, and there are no clinical trials comparing rituximab with cyclophosphamide in this population.

In summary, GI manifestations of rheumatoid vasculitis are exceedingly rare but must be considered in patients with longstanding, seropositive, and erosive RA who present with abdominal pain. Despite an overall decrease in disease incidence, GI disease in rheumatoid vasculitis is associated with a poor prognosis and high rates of mortality.

SECONDARY AMYLOIDOSIS

Secondary (formerly known as "AA") amyloidosis is an uncommon yet important complication of rheumatoid arthritis (33). Longstanding, uncontrolled inflammation leads to the production of pro-inflammatory cytokines such as IL-1, IL-6, and TNF-alpha, resulting in high levels of the acute phase reactant serum amyloid A (SAA) (34). SAA is then cleaved and misfolded into AA amyloid fibrils that deposit in tissues and ultimately disrupt function, leading to a constellation of symptoms known as secondary amyloidosis (35).

Secondary amyloidosis can be due to a variety of chronic inflammatory diseases but is most reported in rheumatoid arthritis. In a report of 374 patients with secondary amyloidosis over 15 years, the majority of patients (33%) had RA (35). Likewise, in a cohort of secondary amyloid from the Netherlands, 56% of cases were due to RA (36). Other diagnoses associated with secondary amyloid include juvenile idiopathic arthritis, chronic sepsis (bronchiectasis, injection drug abuse, osteomyelitis, and tuberculosis), periodic fever syndromes, and Crohn's disease. Like in rheumatoid vasculitis, secondary amyloid tends to present years after diagnosis of RA, with a median duration disease of 15 to 17 years at the time of diagnosis (35, 37).

The incidence of secondary amyloidosis is likely underestimated and is only seen in a small minority of patients for unknown reasons. Prevalence is estimated from 0.6% to 1.1% (38, 39), with estimates of subclinical disease from random fat pad biopsy seen in up to 29% of RA patients (40, 41). Early and aggressive treatment of RA with DMARDs and biologics has reduced the incidence of secondary amyloid (34), much like in rheumatoid vasculitis.

The kidneys are the primary site of deposition of AA amyloid and, classically, can lead to nephrotic syndrome (33). Amyloidosis should be suspected in any patient with rheumatoid arthritis presenting with unexplained renal dysfunction and proteinuria. Gastrointestinal symptoms are varied but common and second only to renal manifestations. Patients with GI disease may present with chronic constipation, diarrhea, malabsorption, and unintentional weight loss (34). Bleeding can also occur due to amyloid deposition in the bowel wall or blood vessels. Patients can also present with hepatomegaly and elevated alkaline phosphatase, but less than a quarter of those patients have hepatic amyloid deposition. Synthetic dysfunction from hepatic amyloid is uncommon (35, 42).

Takeuchi et al. reported the case of a 62-year-old woman with a 16-year history of rheumatoid arthritis and known secondary amyloidosis from a resected gastric polyp 9 years prior. She presented with constipation and was found to have free air on CT of the abdomen, secondary to a perforated rectal diverticulum. She underwent a Hartmann's procedure and was found to have amyloid deposition with Congo red staining in the stroma of the lamina propria mucosa and submucosa of the rectum. The blood vessels lumens were also narrowed due to amyloid deposition (43).

Diagnosis of gastrointestinal disease from secondary amyloid is made on biopsy of the upper or lower GI tract. Central to the management of secondary amyloidosis is control of the underlying RA, which will turn off SAA production.

FELTY'S SYNDROME AND NODULAR REGENERATIVE HYPERPLASIA

Felty's syndrome is a rare complication of rheumatoid arthritis, characterized by the triad of RA, neutropenia, and splenomegaly. It tends to occur in poorly controlled disease associated with nodulosis (44). Nodular regenerative hyperplasia (NRH) is a cause of noncirrhotic portal hypertension that can be seen in rheumatoid arthritis with or without Felty's syndrome. NRH describes a benign transformation of the hepatic parenchyma to small nodules without evidence of fibrosis.

NRH is a slow and progressive disorder that can range from asymptomatic to life-threatening with gastrointestinal bleeding from esophageal varices and ascites requiring frequent paracentesis. Unlike in cirrhosis, measures of synthetic function will be normal, and there will not be stigmata of hyperestrogenism, such as spider angiomata, gynecomastia, or palmar erythema (45).

Diagnosis of NRH is made by liver biopsy but requires reticulin staining and hence a high index of suspicion (45). Management focuses on treatment of the underlying disease, in this case RA, as well as the complications associated with noncirrhotic portal hypertension.

SJOGREN'S DISEASE

Sjogren's disease is characterized by chronic inflammation in the exocrine glands, leading to the cardinal features of dry eyes (keratoconjunctivitis sicca) and dry mouth (xerostomia). It is often designated as primary Sjogren's syndrome (pSS) when no other rheumatic disease is present, though it can also be a secondary finding in RA, lupus, and systemic sclerosis. The diagnosis of Sjogren's is predicated on the presence of clinically significant sicca syndrome as described earlier, positive SSA, and/or SSB antibodies or a salivary gland biopsy showing foci of lymphocytic infiltration.

Many recent advances have been made in furthering our understanding of extraglandular disease, with a focus on interstitial lung disease and the myriad of neurological phenomena in particular. Gastrointestinal manifestations, however, are very common and can adversely impact the patient's quality of life in significant ways. This section will review the variety of GI findings and their direct consequences in patients with pSS as well as the most frequent autoimmune comorbidities.

The Oral Cavity and Esophagus

Xerostomia is one of the hallmark features of Sjogren's and, in many cases, can be severe. The patient may complain of difficulty swallowing dry food, easy sticking of the oral mucosa, and altered taste. Salivary gland enlargement, occasionally painful, can also be seen. Due to the reduced salivary flow, the natural protective effects of saliva are lost with disruption of the oral flora. This can lead to dental caries and oral candidiasis (46). When a patient complains of oral pain, oral infections are highest on the differential, though burning mouth

syndrome is also a common culprit. This describes a diffuse pain throughout the oral cavity in the absence of objective mucosal abnormalities. The etiology of this entity is not clear. However, there are some intriguing data to suggest that it could be driven by a small fiber neuropathy. This may be particularly pertinent if there are other neurological abnormalities on history and physical exam (47).

One downstream effect of oral dryness is dysphagia. However, several studies have shown an inconsistent relationship between swallowing problems and salivary flow measurements, suggesting that additional factors such as GERD or dysmotility might be playing a role in many patients (48). The prevalence of dysphagia in these studies varied widely from 30% to 80%. A prospective cohort study of 4,650 Sjogren's patients found that the risk of gastroesophageal reflux disease for Sjogren's syndrome patients was 2.41-fold greater than that for the comparison cohort after adjusting for age, sex, and comorbidities (49). Chronic cough might therefore be present even in the absence of Sjogren's-associated lung disease.

The Stomach

GI dysmotility may occur distal to the esophagus and cause significant postprandial nausea, which can lead to food avoidance and weight loss in severe cases. Sjogren's disease appears to have a predilection for the peripheral nervous system, with manifestations ranging from dorsal column ganglionitis and vasculitic neuropathy to painful small fiber neuropathy (50). As with burning mouth syndrome, there may be a connection between GI symptoms and neurological pathology. Autoimmune autonomic ganglionopathy (AAG), which can present with a mixture of sympathetic and parasympathetic dysfunction, may affect the gastrointestinal tract with signs of "enteric failure." This could manifest as achalasia, gastroparesis, or ileus. If a patient with Sjogren's has objective findings of a motility disorder such as gastroparesis, it should prompt a review for other features of autonomic dysfunction. In a subset of patients, autoantibodies to the ganglionic acetylcholine receptor may be measurable, though there can be discrepancies between different assays (51). Motility disorders are notoriously challenging to manage, but immune-mediated neuropathy might conceivably represent a therapeutic target, which would render measurement of these antibodies potentially useful. For example, in a small retrospective case series of four patients with pSS and autonomic neuropathy, there was demonstrable improvement in both clinical parameters and autonomic testing following administration of intravenous immunoglobulin in all patients and adjunctive rituximab therapy in one patient (52). Further study, however, is required to see if the symptoms caused by enteric failure are reversible with immune therapies.

Gastritis is another symptom that is more common in patients with connective tissue diseases compared to the general population. Chronic atrophic gastritis may be caused by *H. pylori* infection or, more rarely, autoimmune destruction of the parietal cells lining the gastric mucosa. In many cases, atrophic gastritis can lead to dyspepsia and iron and vitamin B12 deficiencies. The prevalence of antiparietal cell antibodies was described to be as high as 27% in one study of 335 patients with pSS, whereas true atrophic gastritis was seen in approximately 2% (53). It is conceivable that this number would be higher if the patients with positive antibodies were followed prospectively over several years.

Sjogren's and the Gut

A burgeoning area of research is the relationship between the gut microbiome and autoimmune diseases, and Sjogren's is no exception to this trend. Diminished secretions may compromise the integrity of the gut epithelium and its barrier function and alter the natural flora, leading to intestinal dysbiosis (imbalance of microorganisms). Intestinal dysbiosis has been reported both in mouse models of pSS and in patients, with a correlation in the murine model with more severe sicca syndrome (54). In a series of 42 pSS patients compared to 35 age- and sex-matched controls, there was an increased prevalence of severe dysbiosis affecting 21% of the patient sample (55). Milder levels of micro-organism imbalance were present in both groups, illustrating the diversity of these microbial signatures in the normal population. There was an association with higher levels of fecal calprotectin and higher clinical scores of Sjogren's disease activity but, interestingly, no correlation with either inflammatory bowel disease or the more common irritable bowel syndrome.

Table 3.1 Summarizes the Varied GI findings in Patients with pSS

Gastrointestinal Complications of Sjogren's (In Order of Frequency)	
Oral cavity	Xerostomia
	Burning mouth syndrome
	Candidiasis
Esophagus	Dysphagia
	GERD
	Esophageal dysmotility
Stomach	Atrophic gastritis
	Gastroparesis
Bowel	Constipation
	Microscopic colitis
	Cryoglobulinemic vasculitis

Constipation is a frequent finding in patients with Sjogren's disease, but other colonic complications are uncommon. Microscopic colitis is characterized by chronic, watery diarrhea in patients with normal macroscopic findings on endoscopy but abnormal histopathology. The disease can be further divided into an either lymphocytic or collagenous subtype. Concomitant autoimmunity is seen in around a third of patients, but celiac disease and thyroiditis are the strongest associations (56). Of the 16.2% of pSS patients in a Spanish cohort with digestive involvement, 4.2% were diagnosed with lymphocytic colitis (57). Sjogren's disease can also be associated with a type III mixed cryoglobulinemia, well recognized to cause cutaneous and neurological findings. However, ischemic colitis related to vasculitis in Sjogren's remains very rare, and evaluation for concomitant hypercoagulability should be sought in such cases (58). Table 3.1 summarizes the various effects of Sjogren's in the gastrointestinal system.

LIVER DISEASE

Primary biliary cholangitis (PBC) describes lymphocytic infiltration of the small intralobular bile ducts, damaging the epithelial cells and leading to their eventual obliteration. Many patients are diagnosed following the incidental discovery of cholestatic changes in blood tests, but if left undetected, the disease will cause pruritus, fatigue, and eventual signs of advanced liver disease such as ascites and jaundice. In the past, cirrhosis would have been a frequent sequela of cholestasis, but with the widespread use of ursodeoxycholic acid, this is now uncommon. This prompted the change in nomenclature from primary biliary cirrhosis.

There are striking parallels in the pathophysiology of Sjogren's disease and PBC. At a cellular level, the lymphocytic infiltration and eventual breakdown of the bile ducts and exocrine glands are mirrored, leading to the theory that these entities exist on a spectrum of "autoimmune epithelitis" (59), as shown in Figure 3.1 and Figure 3.2. In terms of clinical similarities, both diseases strongly

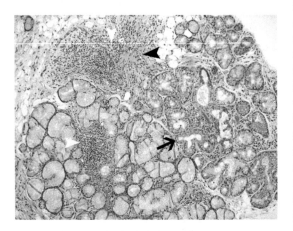

Figure 3.1 This is an H&E image at 100x magnification of a minor salivary gland lobule of the lip. There are foci of chronic inflammation (white arrowheads), fibrosis (black arrowhead), and relative flattening of the acinar epithelial cells, consistent with atrophy (black arrow). Attr: N Cipriani, University of Chicago Pathology.

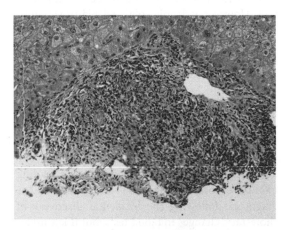

Figure 3.2 This is a histopathology slide from a patient with primary biliary cholangitis illustrating dense lymphocytic infiltrate and bile duct atrophy. Attr: R Anders, John Hopkins Pathology.

favor women by an estimated 10:1 ratio and are more common in middle age. Antimitochondrial antibodies, which are the serological hallmark of PBC, are estimated to occur in up to 20% of patients with pSS even in the absence of liver abnormalities, though with direct immunofluorescence, this number may be closer to 5.1% (59).

The exact degree of association or coexistence between these two diseases is disputed. A medical record review of 1,554 patients with PBC detected extrahepatic autoimmune disease at a rate of 28.3% (60). Autoimmune thyroid diseases were the most common (10.6%), but Sjogren's disease (8.3%) was next, with other connective tissue diseases such as scleroderma and lupus occurring at a much lower frequency. The rate of sicca syndrome in PBC may be higher yet, without serological findings or salivary gland biopsy necessarily present to confirm SS (61). Conversely, in a Portuguese center, a retrospective review of 115 patients with pSS found a prevalence of PBC of 5.2% (62). This small difference may be because pSS is a more common diagnosis than PBC. Sjogren's syndrome has an incidence of approximately 6.9 per 100,000 person-years versus 2.7 per 100,000 person-years for PBC (63, 64).

Autoimmune hepatitis (AIH) is a chronic inflammatory disease of the liver characterized by abnormal levels of serum globulins, circulating autoantibodies, and histological findings of periportal or interface hepatitis. The most commonly associated antibodies include antinuclear antibodies and anti-smooth muscle antibody, but additional serological markers such as antiliver kidney microsomal-1 and atypical perinuclear antineutrophil cytoplasmic antibody (p-ANCA) can be seen. The disease is responsive to immunosuppression with steroids and azathioprine or mycophenolate mofetil in up to 80% of patients, so early detection and diagnosis are desirable to prevent the development of fibrosis (65). It is interesting that variants of AIH have been described that overlap with PBC, so hybrid pathology is not unusual. The prevalence of AIH in a John Hopkins cohort of 58 patients with primary Sjogren's syndrome (pSS) was 1.7%, which is consistent with an estimated 1% to 4% in multiple other series (66). Therefore, this is a weaker association than seen with PBC, but it remains higher than the normal population.

It is important to note that the most common cause of abnormal liver function tests in patients with pSS is nonalcoholic fatty liver disease, just as in the general population (67). However, as we have argued in this chapter, the index of suspicion for an autoimmune pathology should be higher when Sjogren's disease is present. Depending on the pattern of abnormalities, further investigation may involve additional autoantibody testing to look for either autoimmune hepatitis or PBC, with imaging and need for liver biopsy to be determined after consultation with a liver specialist. It is noteworthy that patients with Sjogren's disease who have positive mitochondrial antibodies develop symptomatic PBC at a high rate and typically within a 5-year follow-up period (68). Early and regular screening for these autoantibodies could therefore be justified as part of the comprehensive care of a patient with Sjogren's disease, regardless of the presence of liver chemistry abnormalities.

CONCLUSION

Gastrointestinal disease in RA is uncommon but can be due to rheumatoid vasculitis, secondary amyloidosis, and Felty's syndrome with nodular regenerative hyperplasia. These entities occur most often in patients with longstanding, seropositive, and erosive RA. Central to prevention of these complications is early and aggressive disease control. Meanwhile, GI manifestations secondary to Sjogren's disease can present at any time along the disease course, with the potential for overlap with autoimmune gastroenterological conditions such as primary biliary cholangitis, autoimmune hepatitis, and atrophic gastritis. Further study is recommended to improve understanding of the pathophysiology of the GI manifestations of these two common rheumatic diseases so that better outcomes can be sought for the patient.

REFERENCES

1. Allison MC, Howatson AG, Torrance CJ et al. Gastrointestinal damage associated with the use of nonsteroidal antiinflammatory drugs. N Engl J Med. 1992 Sep 10;327(11):749–54.
2. Bannatyne GA. Rheumatoid arthritis: Its pathology, morbid anatomy, and treatment. 2nd ed. Bristol: John Wright & Co.; 1898.
3. Bywaters EG, Scott JT. The natural history of vascular lesions in rheumatoid arthritis. J Chronic Dis. 1963 Aug;16:905–14.
4. Myasoedova E, Crowson CS, Turesson C et al. Incidence of extraarticular rheumatoid arthritis in Olmsted County, Minnesota, in 1995–2007 versus 1985–1994: A population-based study. J Rheumatol. 2011 Jun;38(6):983–9.
5. Watts RA, Carruthers DM, Symmons DP et al. The incidence of rheumatoid vasculitis in the Norwich Health Authority. Br J Rheumatol. 1994 Sep;33(9):832–3.
6. Ntatsaki E, Mooney J, Scott DGI et al. Systemic rheumatoid vasculitis in the era of modern immunosuppressive therapy. Rheumatol (Oxford). 2014 Jan;53(1):145–52.
7. Makol A, Matteson EL, Warrington KJ. Rheumatoid vasculitis: An update. Curr Opin Rheumatol. 2015 Jan;27(1):63–70.
8. Grigor C, Capell H, Stirling A et al. Effect of a treatment strategy of tight control for rheumatoid arthritis (the TICORA study): A single-blind randomised controlled trial. Lancet. 2004;364(9430):263–9.
9. Scott DG, Bacon PA. Intravenous cyclophosphamide plus methylprednisolone in treatment of systemic rheumatoid vasculitis. Am J Med. 1984 Mar;76(3):377–84.
10. Voskuyl AE, Zwinderman AH, Westedt ML et al. Factors associated with the development of vasculitis in rheumatoid arthritis: Results of a case-control study. Ann Rheum Dis. 1996 Mar;55(3):190–2.
11. Mongan ES, Cass RM, Jacox RF et al. A study of the relation of seronegative and seropositive rheumatoid arthritis to each other and to necrotizing vasculitis. Am J Med. 1969 Jul;47(1):23–35.
12. Makol A, Crowson CS, Wetter DA et al. Vasculitis associated with rheumatoid arthritis: A case-control study. Rheumatol (Oxford). 2014 May;53(5):890–9.
13. Turesson C, Jacobsson LTH, Matteson EL. Cardiovascular comorbidity in rheumatic diseases. Vasc Health Risk Manag. 2008;4(3):605–14.
14. Puéchal X, Said G, Hilliquin P et al. Peripheral neuropathy with necrotizing vasculitis in rheumatoid arthritis: A clinicopathologic and prognostic study of

thirty-two patients. *Arthritis Rheum.* 1995 Nov;38(11):1618–29.

15. Babian M, Nasef S, Soloway G. Gastrointestinal infarction as a manifestation of rheumatoid vasculitis. *Am J Gastroenterol.* 1998 Jan;93(1):119–20.

16. Marcolongo R, Bayeli PF, Montagnani M. Gastrointestinal involvement in rheumatoid arthritis: A biopsy study. *J Rheumatol.* 1979;6(2):163–73.

17. Lee SY, Lee SW, Chung WT. Jejunal vasculitis in patient with rheumatoid arthritis: Case report and literature review. *Mod Rheumatol.* 2012 Nov;22(6):924–7.

18. Parker B, Chattopadhyay C. A case of rheumatoid vasculitis involving the gastrointestinal tract in early disease. *Rheumatol (Oxford).* 2007 Nov;46(11):1737–8.

19. Burt RW, Berenson MM, Samuelson CO et al. Rheumatoid vasculitis of the colon presenting as pancolitis. *Dig Dis Sci.* 1983 Feb;28(2):183–8.

20. Scott DG, Bacon PA, Tribe CR. Systemic rheumatoid vasculitis: A clinical and laboratory study of 50 cases. *Med.* 1981 Jul;60(4):288–97.

21. Mosley JG, Desai A, Gupta I. Mesenteric arteritis. *Gut.* 1990 Aug;31(8):956–7.

22. Jacobsen SE, Petersen P, Jensen P. Acute abdomen in rheumatoid arthritis due to mesenteric arteritis: A case report and review. *Dan Med Bull.* 1985 Jun;32(3):191–3.

23. Geirsson AJ, Sturfelt G, Truedsson L. Clinical and serological features of severe vasculitis in rheumatoid arthritis: Prognostic implications. *Ann Rheum Dis.* 1987 Oct;46(10):727–33.

24. Kuehne SE, Gauvin GP, Shortsleeve MJ. Small bowel stricture caused by rheumatoid vasculitis. *Radiology.* 1992 Jul;184(1):215–16.

25. Tago M, Naito Y, Aihara H et al. Recurrent stenosis of the ileum caused by rheumatoid vasculitis. *Intern Med.* 2016;55(7):819–23.

26. van Laar JM, Smit VT, de Beus WM et al. Rheumatoid vasculitis presenting as appendicitis. *Clin Exp Rheumatol.* 1998;16(6):736–8.

27. Mizuno K, Ikeda K, Saida Y et al. Hepatic hemorrhage in malignant rheumatoid arthritis. *Am J Gastroenterol.* 1996 Dec;91(12):2624–5.

28. Achkar AA, Stanson AW, Johnson CM et al. Rheumatoid vasculitis manifesting as intra-abdominal hemorrhage. *Mayo Clin Proc.* 1995 Jun;70(6):565–9.

29. Jayawardene SA, Sheerin N, Pattison JM et al. Spontaneous abdominal hemorrhage with AA-amyloidosis and vasculitis in a patient with rheumatoid arthritis. *J Clin Rheumatol.* 2001 Apr;7(2):86–90.

30. Pagnoux C, Mahr A, Cohen P et al. Presentation and outcome of gastrointestinal involvement in systemic necrotizing vasculitides: Analysis of 62 patients with polyarteritis nodosa, microscopic polyangiitis, Wegener granulomatosis, Churg-Strauss syndrome, or rheumatoid arthritis-associated vasculitis. *Med.* 2005 Mar;84(2):115–28.

31. Tsai JT. Perforation of the small bowel with rheumatoid arthritis. *South Med J.* 1980 Jul;73(7):939–40.

32. Puéchal X, Gottenberg JE, Berthelot JM et al. Rituximab therapy for systemic vasculitis associated with rheumatoid arthritis: Results from the AutoImmunity and Rituximab Registry. *Arthritis Care Res (Hoboken).* 2012 Mar;64(3):331–9.

33. Nakamura T. Clinical strategies for amyloid A amyloidosis secondary to rheumatoid arthritis. *Mod Rheumatol.* 2008;18(2):109–18.

34. Girnius S, Dember L, Doros G et al. The changing face of AA amyloidosis: A single center experience. *Amyloid.* 2011 Jun;18(Suppl 1):226–8.

35. Lachmann HJ, Goodman HJB, Gilbertson JA et al. Natural history and outcome in systemic AA amyloidosis. *N Engl J Med.* 2007 Jun 7;356(23):2361–71.

36. Hazenberg BP, van Rijswijk MH. Clinical and therapeutic aspects of AA amyloidosis. *Baillieres Clin Rheumatol.* 1994 Aug;8(3):661–90.

37. Husby G. Amyloidosis. *Semin Arthritis Rheum.* 1992 Oct;22(2):67–82.

38. Carmona L, González-Alvaro I, Balsa A et al. Rheumatoid arthritis in Spain: Occurrence of extra-articular manifestations and estimates of disease severity. *Ann Rheum Dis.* 2003 Sep;62(9):897–900.

39. Calgüneri M, Ureten K, Akif Oztürk M et al. Extra-articular manifestations of rheumatoid

arthritis: Results of a university hospital of 526 patients in Turkey. *Clin Exp Rheumatol.* 2006;24(3):305–8.

40. Wiland P, Wojtala R, Goodacre J et al. The prevalence of subclinical amyloidosis in Polish patients with rheumatoid arthritis. *Clin Rheumatol.* 2004 Jun;23(3):193–8.

41. El Mansoury TM, Hazenberg BPC, El Badawy SA et al. Screening for amyloid in subcutaneous fat tissue of Egyptian patients with rheumatoid arthritis: Clinical and laboratory characteristics. *Ann Rheum Dis.* 2002 Jan;61(1):42–7.

42. Gertz MA, Kyle RA. Secondary systemic amyloidosis: Response and survival in 64 patients. *Med.* 1991 Jul;70(4):246–56.

43. Takeuchi D, Koide N, Kitazawa M et al. Perforation of rectal diverticulum with amyloidosis secondary to rheumatoid arthritis: Case report and review of the literature. *Clin J Gastroenterol.* 2010 Feb;3(1):30–5.

44. Craig E, Cappelli LC. Gastrointestinal and hepatic disease in rheumatoid arthritis. *Rheum Dis Clin North Am.* 2018 Feb;44(1):89–111.

45. Jain P, Patel S, Simpson HN et al. Nodular regenerative hyperplasia of the liver in rheumatic disease: Cases and review of the literature. *J Investig Med High Impact Case Rep.* 2021;9:23247096211044616.

46. Soto-Rojas AE, Villa AR, Sifuentes-Osornio J et al. Oral manifestations in patients with Sjögren's syndrome. *J Rheumatol.* 1998 May;25(5):906–10.

47. Jääskeläinen SK. Is burning mouth syndrome a neuropathic pain condition? *Pain.* 2018 Mar;159(3):610–13.

48. Ebert EC. Gastrointestinal and hepatic manifestations of Sjogren syndrome. *J Clin Gastroenterol.* 2012 Jan;46(1):25–30.

49. Chang CS, Liao CH, Muo CH et al. Increased risk of concurrent gastroesophageal reflux disease among patients with Sjögren's syndrome: A nationwide population-based study. *Eur J Intern Med.* 2016 Jun;31:73–8.

50. Chai J, Logigian EL. Neurological manifestations of primary Sjogren's syndrome. *Curr Opin Neurol.* 2010 Oct;23(5):509–13.

51. Urriola N, Adelstein S. Autoimmune autonomic ganglionopathy: Ganglionic acetylcholine receptor autoantibodies. *Autoimmun Rev.* 2022 Feb;21(2):102988.

52. Goodman BP. Immunoresponsive autonomic neuropathy in Sjögren syndrome- case series and literature review. *Am J Ther.* 2019;26(1):e66–71.

53. Nardi N, Brito-Zerón P, Ramos-Casals M et al. Circulating auto-antibodies against nuclear and non-nuclear antigens in primary Sjögren's syndrome: Prevalence and clinical significance in 335 patients. *Clin Rheumatol.* 2006 May;25(3):341–6.

54. de Paiva CS, Jones DB, Stern ME et al. Altered mucosal microbiome diversity and disease severity in Sjögren syndrome. *Sci Rep.* 2016 Apr 18;6:23561.

55. Mandl T, Marsal J, Olsson P et al. Severe intestinal dysbiosis is prevalent in primary Sjögren's syndrome and is associated with systemic disease activity. *Arthritis Res Ther.* 2017 Oct 24;19(1):237.

56. Kao KT, Pedraza BA, McClune AC et al. Microscopic colitis: A large retrospective analysis from a health maintenance organization experience. *World J Gastroenterol.* 2009 Jul 7;15(25):3122–7.

57. Melchor S, Sánchez-Piedra C, Fernández Castro M et al. Digestive involvement in primary Sjögren's syndrome: Analysis from the Sjögrenser registry. *Clin Exp Rheumatol.* 2020;38(Suppl 126, 4):110–15.

58. Boukadida K. Challenging case of ischemic colitis, necrotic cutaneous vasculitis and thromboembolic disease in an elderly patient with Sjogren's syndrome. *Oxf Med Case Rep.* 2019 Nov;2019(11):464–5.

59. Colapietro F, Lleo A, Generali E. Antimitochondrial antibodies: From bench to bedside. *Clin Rev Allergy Immunol.* 2022 Oct;63(2):166–77.

60. Efe C, Torgutalp M, Henriksson I et al. Extrahepatic autoimmune diseases in primary biliary cholangitis: Prevalence and significance for clinical presentation and disease outcome. *J Gastroenterol Hepatol.* 2021 Apr;36(4):936–42.

61. Selmi C, Meroni PL, Gershwin ME. Primary biliary cirrhosis and Sjögren's syndrome: Autoimmune epithelitis. *J Autoimmun.* 2012 Aug;39(1–2):34–42.

62. Santos GA, Brandão M, Farinha F. Prevalence of primary biliary cholangitis in a cohort of primary Sjögren's syndrome patients. *Cureus.* 2022 Apr;14(4):e24590.

63. Qin B, Wang J, Yang Z et al. Epidemiology of primary Sjögren's syndrome: A systematic review and meta-analysis. *Ann Rheum Dis*. 2015 Nov;74(11):1983–9.

64. Kim WR, Lindor KD, Locke GR et al. Epidemiology and natural history of primary biliary cirrhosis in a US community. *Gastroenterol*. 2000 Dec;119(6):1631–6.

65. Krawitt EL. Autoimmune hepatitis. *N Engl J Med*. 2006 Jan 5;354(1):54–66.

66. Karp JK, Akpek EK, Anders RA. Autoimmune hepatitis in patients with primary Sjögren's syndrome: A series of two-hundred and two patients. *Int J Clin Exp Pathol*. 2010 Mar 25;3(6):582–6.

67. Sun Y, Zhang W, Li B et al. The coexistence of Sjögren's syndrome and primary biliary cirrhosis: A comprehensive review. *Clin Rev Allergy Immunol*. 2015 Jun;48(2–3):301–15.

68. Csepregi A, Szodoray P, Zeher M. Do autoantibodies predict autoimmune liver disease in primary Sjögren's syndrome? Data of 180 patients upon a 5 year follow-up. *Scand J Immunol*. 2002 Dec;56(6):623–9.

4

Ankylosing Spondylitis and Psoriatic Arthritis

REEM JAN

SPONDYLOARTHRITIS

Spondyloarthritis (SpA) is a broad category of diseases that encompass characteristic spinal findings (axial SpA) and inflammatory changes in the large joints, tendon/ligament insertion sites (enthesitis), or an entire digit (dactylitis). This distinction between axial and peripheral disease is important for therapeutic considerations, but patients can present anywhere along the spectrum of these clinical manifestations. Axial SpA in its most severe form is also known as ankylosing spondylitis, defined by bilateral sacroiliitis detectable on plain radiographs. These patients are at particular risk for spinal fusion and deformities. Both axial and peripheral SpA can be associated with anterior uveitis, psoriasis, or inflammatory bowel disease or occur as an immunological reaction to recent gastrointestinal or genitourinary infection (reactive arthritis). In this chapter, we will focus on ankylosing spondylitis and psoriatic arthritis as prototypical examples of this group of disorders and discuss associated gastrointestinal complications.

AXIAL SPONDYLOARTHRITIS

It is important for the physician to be able to identify high-risk features of back pain and appropriately triage the patients that require further evaluation for axial SpA. This is rendered challenging by the high frequency of back pain complaints in primary care and the relative scarcity of cases of true inflammatory disease. The prevalence of axial SpA ranges from 0.02% in Sub-Saharan Africa to 0.35% in Northern Arctic communities (1). Delay to diagnosis can therefore be unacceptably prolonged for many patients, with a large metanalysis reporting a mean delay of 6.7 years (2).

Inflammatory back pain is the hallmark of axial SpA. In 2009, the Assessment of Spondyloarthritis International Society (ASAS) ultimately determined that the following features were the most discriminating (3):

- Age of onset < 40 years
- Insidious onset
- Improvement with exercise
- No improvement with rest
- Pain at night (with improvement upon awakening)

However, it must be noted that inflammatory back pain does not consistently correlate with a subsequent diagnosis of axial SpA. Both the sensitivity and specificity are far enhanced when other supportive findings are added to the diagnostic criteria (4). These may include HLA-B27 positivity, history of inflammatory bowel disease, psoriasis, or uveitis and clinical response to nonsteroidal anti-inflammatory drugs.

Our understanding of the epidemiology of axial SpA has changed with the use of magnetic resonance imaging (MRI) to detect sacroiliitis. This has given rise to a subcategory of disease designated as

DOI: 10.1201/9781003367307-4

nonradiographic axial SpA. These patients are at lower risk for structural damage and have a more equal sex distribution and a weaker association with HLA-B27 (5). Radiographic axial SpA, on the other hand, is more likely to follow the natural history of ankylosing spondylitis: bilateral sacroiliac inflammation that progresses caudally up the spine if untreated, with syndesmophyte formation and slow fusion of the axial skeleton.

First-line treatment of axial SpA is non-steroidal anti-inflammatory drugs (NSAID), which aim to alleviate stiffness and pain and improve function. It remains controversial whether daily long-term use significantly impacts radiographic progression, but this may be limited in any event by the potential toxicity of this approach. TNF inhibitors have shown excellent outcomes for symptom management, and there is some evidence that they reduce spinal radiographic progression (6). IL-17A inhibitors and JAK inhibitors are now also approved for nonradiographic and nonradiographic axial SpA, and comparative studies are underway to help improve patient selection and treatment algorithm approaches. Physical therapy and exercise remain integral to the management of all patients with axial SpA.

PSORIATIC ARTHRITIS

Psoriasis is a chronic inflammatory skin condition characterized by the formation of exfoliative well-circumscribed erythematous plaques with a predilection for the scalp, ears, and extensor surfaces of joints. More challenging subtypes include nail pitting and dystrophy, palmar-plantar psoriasis, and lesions that favor the skin folds (inverse psoriasis). All these subtypes may be associated with inflammatory arthritis. Psoriatic arthritis (PsA) is estimated to occur in about 30% of patients with psoriasis and can lead to significant morbidity (7).

Dactylitis is one of the most common manifestations of PsA, occurring in 40% to 50% of patients. It describes swelling and inflammation of an entire digit due to tenosynovitis and soft tissue edema. The third and fourth toes are peculiarly affected, but the fingers can also be involved. It is associated with higher risk of bone erosions and new bone formation (8). Figure 4.1 shows a classic case of dactylitis. Enthesitis follows the same pattern in all peripheral SpA, with the Achilles tendon and plantar fascia highly favored; additional

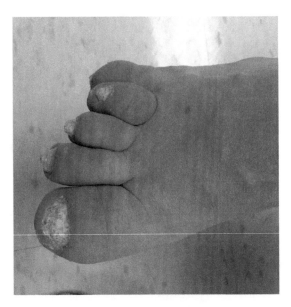

Figure 4.1 Dactylitis in first and fourth toes.

sites include the patella, iliac crest, epicondyles, and supraspinatus insertions (9). PsA, however is unique in its ability to cause inflammatory arthritis at the distal interphalangeal joints (DIP), and this is intimately associated with the presence of nail disease (Figure 4.2).

Axial PsA may represent its own disease entity, as there are some key distinctions from traditional paradigms of axial SpA. Sacroiliitis is more likely to be unilateral, and nonmarginal syndesmophytes may form as the disease progresses, leading to a less severe phenotype than ankylosing spondylitis. Importantly, there is earlier involvement of the cervical spine that includes risk of facet fusion, and this can occur in the absence of sacroiliac disease (10). Including these patients in clinical trials will help us understand if they respond to a wider range of biologic therapy than axial SpA.

AXIAL SPONDYLOARTHRITIS AND THE BOWEL

The bowels are more than a digestive organ; they act as a living part of the immune system, a reservoir of millions of microorganisms that are unique in composition between individuals. We have long understood that infectious processes in the GI tract can trigger immune-mediated inflammatory events in other areas of the body, such as Guillain–Barré syndrome following dysentery. In the field of

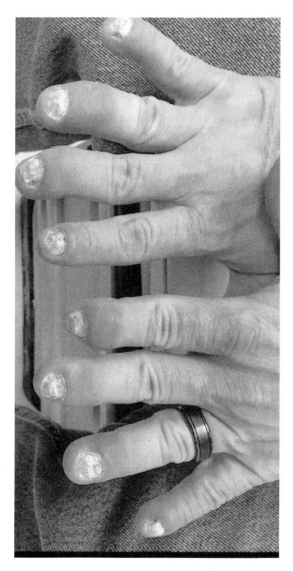

Figure 4.2 Psoriatic nail disease with DIP arthritis.

rheumatology, reactive arthritis describes a sterile inflammatory arthritis that occurs in response to a gastrointestinal or genitourinary infection, most frequently *Yersinia*, *Campylobacter*, *Shigella*, and *Chlamydia*. This pattern of arthritis closely allies with other clinical entities in the spondyloarthritis family, with manifestations that include asymmetric oligoarthritis, enthesitis, dactylitis, and sacroiliitis. Anywhere between 5% and 10% of patients with Crohn's and ulcerative colitis have axial SpA, and higher numbers are cited for peripheral joint inflammation.

Drawing upon this model, it has been postulated that gut inflammation is an important etiological factor in the development of axial spondyloarthritis. Ileocolonoscopies demonstrate more frequent endoscopic lesions in patients with spondylarthritis (44%) compared with those with other inflammatory joint diseases (6%; $p = 0.001$), and this is not associated with NSAID use (11). In the absence of macroscopic pathology, histological evaluation and immunohistochemistry has shown an increased number of lymphoid follicles in both the ileum ($p < 0.01$) and the colon ($p < 0.01$) of SpA patients compared to controls (12). Although histological gut inflammation at initial scope is associated with progression of arthritis, evolution to inflammatory bowel disease remains uncommon. De Vos et al. found that 7% of SpA patients with initial endoscopic assessment progressed to clinically apparent bowel disease (at a median of 70-month follow-up period) (13). Routine endoscopic evaluation for inflammatory bowel disease is not recommended for patients with axial SpA in the absence of any gastrointestinal symptoms (14). Conversely, there is a high degree of asymptomatic sacroiliitis detected on imaging in patients with Crohn's disease (15). In such cases, the HLA-B27 association is weaker than in clinical axial SpA, and other genetic factors such as CARD15 may be more relevant (16). Further study is required to determine whether these patients will develop more inflammatory back pain as time progresses.

There is unlikely to be a linear relationship between gut inflammation and axial or joint disease in SpA. This complexity is highlighted by the "tissue-based compartmentalization" of IL-17 and related cytokines such as IL-23 in the pathogenesis of spine, joint, skin, and bowel inflammation (17). While IL-17A has proven to be an effective target for the treatment of ankylosing spondylitis and psoriatic arthritis, blockade of this cytokine both promotes IBD flares and can unmask previously silent or de novo bowel inflammation. The incidence of Crohn's and ulcerative colitis in this setting remains fairly low at 2.4 per 1,000 patient-years but nonetheless merits careful patient selection for IL-17A inhibition and long-term monitoring (18). Genome-wide associated studies have demonstrated single nucleotide polymorphisms in the IL-23R pathway across the spectrum of seronegative spondyloarthritides, including axial SpA, psoriasis and Crohn's disease (19). This pivotal role for IL-23 is an attractive concept in SpA because enthesitis is thought to be central to the pathophysiology of the sacroiliac and peripheral joint disease, and murine models have shown resident IL-23R expressing myeloid cells in the enthesis (20). In fact, in these studies, the in vivo expression of IL-23 is sufficient to phenocopy the human disease. Disappointingly, IL-23 inhibition through ustekinumab or the p19-specific risankizumab failed to meet outcomes in axial SpA despite excellent results in psoriasis, Crohn's, ulcerative colitis, and psoriatic arthritis.

The intersection between the bowel, spine, eyes, joint, and skin remains an exciting avenue for research because spondyloarthritis draws together several diseases with profound commonalities as well as differences. Elucidating the exact nature and direction of these relationships will enhance our understanding of the mechanisms of disease development and progression and open up new concepts in treatment.

PSORIASIS AND THE LIVER

In the past couple of decades, there has been growing awareness that inflammation interplays with many chronic disease states including cardiovascular disease, obesity, and metabolic syndrome. Superimposed on this association, further evidence points to chronic inflammatory diseases such as rheumatoid arthritis and psoriasis independently increasing the risk for coronary events (21).

Psoriasis represents a unique model to study these relationships. There has been consistent demonstration of a higher prevalence of obesity, cardiovascular disease, diabetes, hyperlipidemia, and NAFLD in patients with psoriasis (22). Some have advocated for considering psoriasis a multiorgan disease (23). In this chapter, we will focus on the liver and, in particular, NAFLD as a manifestation of this.

History shows that patients with psoriasis have been subject to more stringent methotrexate drug monitoring by dermatologists than patients with rheumatic disease. This once involved surveillance liver biopsies for detection of drug-induced fibrosis, an invasive practice that has largely been replaced by frequent lab test monitoring. The question is what does the high detection rate of liver abnormalities truly represent? The simplest explanation is that more aggressive drug monitoring inevitably leads to earlier and more frequent identification of aberrancies. However, several investigators have tried to tease out a tighter association.

A large cohort study compared patients with psoriasis, PsA, and RA with matched controls for incident liver disease and found a stronger association with liver abnormalities in the first two groups (24). This held particularly true for NAFLD and cirrhosis, which increased in a stepwise fashion with increased severity of skin disease (measured by body surface area). A more recent study specifically examined thousands of patients in a Danish health registry receiving methotrexate (5,676 psoriasis; 6,520 PsA; 28,030 RA) and found that this higher rate of liver disease continued to be statistically significant independent of diabetes, hyperlipidemia, and average weekly methotrexate dose (25). BMI, however, was not included in the analysis. Patients with any type of psoriatic disease, therefore, were likely to have shorter duration of exposure to this medication.

Other large-population studies have reinforced this association between psoriasis and NAFLD, and the question remains whether this is a process independent of metabolic comorbidities. A US cross-sectional study using NHANES data found a 42.4% prevalence of NAFLD (defined by the US fatty liver index [USFLI] score) in patients with psoriasis (26). The analysis again adjusted for multiple demographic data inclusive of diabetes and metabolic syndrome. The authors argue that this relationship between psoriasis and NAFLD may therefore be bidirectional. Proinflammatory cytokines upregulated in the lymphocytes and keratinocytes of psoriasis patients may directly contribute to NAFLD development. IL-22 (produced by TH17 cells) and IL-23 have been implicated in a mouse model in the pathogenesis of acanthosis, which is a marker for metabolic disease and NAFLD (27). TNF-alpha has also been shown to induce insulin resistance (28).

Obesity is a frequent comorbidity in many patients with psoriatic disease and undoubtedly exacerbates these tensions. The silver lining is that weight reduction might be of benefit in this population on multiple fronts. In a study of patients with psoriatic arthritis who had a BMI > 33 kg/m^2, weight loss through a very-low-energy diet led to significantly improved disease activity scores based on 28 joint count and CRP (DAS28CRP) (29). The weight loss was also associated with improved levels of serum lipids, glucose, and urate. White adipose tissue secretes a multitude of bioactive peptides that include TNF-alpha, IL-17, IL-23, and leptin; Landgren and colleagues have shown that weight loss in psoriatic arthritis strongly correlates with reduced IL-23 levels and leptin, with TNF-alpha lowered in both PsA and control groups (30). Hence, interventions to address metabolic syndrome and NAFLD, whether through lifestyle or weight-loss medications or surgery, should also impact psoriatic disease outcomes.

CONCLUSION

Spondyloarthritis encompasses a range of fascinating diseases with the potential to manifest inflammation in the spine, enthesitis, joints, and digits but also skin, eyes, and bowel. Further study is required to understand the cause and effect of bowel inflammation in SpA and the myriad organ effects of these systemic inflammatory diseases.

REFERENCES

1. Stolwijk C, van Onna M, Boonen A et al. Global prevalence of spondyloarthritis: A systematic review and meta-regression analysis. *Arthritis Care Res* (Hoboken). 2016 Sep;68(9):1320–31.
2. Zhao SS, Pittam B, Harrison NL et al. Diagnostic delay in axial spondyloarthritis: A systematic review and meta-analysis. *Rheumatol* (Oxford). 2021 Apr 6;60(4):1620–8.
3. Sieper J, van der Heijde D, Landewé R et al. New criteria for inflammatory back pain in patients with chronic back pain: A real patient exercise by experts from the Assessment of SpondyloArthritis International Society (ASAS). *Ann Rheum Dis*. 2009 Jun;68(6):784–8.
4. Weisman MH. Inflammatory back pain: The United States perspective. *Rheum Dis Clin North Am*. 2012 Aug;38(3):501–12.
5. Benavent D, Navarro-Compán V. Understanding the paradigm of non-radiographic axial spondyloarthritis. *Clin Rheumatol*. 2021 Feb;40(2):501–12.
6. Molnar C, Scherer A, Baraliakos X et al. TNF blockers inhibit spinal radiographic progression in ankylosing spondylitis by reducing disease activity: Results from the Swiss Clinical Quality Management cohort. *Ann Rheum Dis*. 2018 Jan;77(1):63–9.
7. Ritchlin CT, Colbert RA, Gladman DD. Psoriatic arthritis. *N Engl J Med*. 2017 Mar 9;376(10):957–70. Erratum in: *N Engl J Med*. 2017 May 25;376(21):2097.
8. Brockbank JE, Stein M, Schentag CT et al. Dactylitis in psoriatic arthritis: A marker for disease severity? *Ann Rheum Dis*. 2005 Feb;64(2):188–90.
9. Kehl AS, Corr M, Weisman MH. Review: Enthesitis: New insights into pathogenesis, diagnostic modalities, and treatment. *Arthritis Rheumatol*. 2016 Feb;68(2):312–22.
10. Poddubnyy D, Jadon DR, Van den Bosch F et al. Axial involvement in psoriatic arthritis: An update for rheumatologists. *Semin Arthritis Rheum*. 2021 Aug;51(4):880–7.
11. Leirisalo-Repo M, Turunen U, Stenman S et al. High frequency of silent inflammatory bowel disease in spondylarthropathy. *Arthritis Rheum*. 1994 Jan;37(1):23–31.
12. Demetter P, Van Huysse JA, De Keyser F et al. Increase in lymphoid follicles and leukocyte adhesion molecules emphasizes a role for the gut in spondyloarthropathy pathogenesis. *J Pathol*. 2002 Dec;198(4):517–22.
13. De Vos M, Mielants H, Cuvelier C et al. Long-term evolution of gut inflammation in patients with spondyloarthropathy. *Gastroenterol*. 1996 Jun;110(6):1696–703.
14. Rudwaleit M, Baeten D. Ankylosing spondylitis and bowel disease. *Best Pract Res Clin Rheumatol*. 2006 Jun;20(3):451–71.
15. Cereser L, Zancan G, Giovannini I et al. Asymptomatic sacroiliitis detected by magnetic resonance enterography in patients with Crohn's disease: Prevalence, association with clinical data, and reliability among radiologists in a multicenter study of adult and pediatric population. *Clin Rheumatol*. 2022 Aug;41(8):2499–511.
16. Peeters H, Vander Cruyssen B, Laukens D et al. Radiological sacroiliitis, a hallmark of spondylitis, is linked with CARD15 gene polymorphisms in patients with Crohn's disease. *Ann Rheum Dis*. 2004 Sep;63(9):1131–4.
17. Gracey E, Vereecke L, McGovern D et al. Revisiting the gut—Joint axis: Links between gut inflammation and spondyloarthritis. *Nat Rev Rheumatol*. 2020;16:415–33.

18. Fauny M, Moulin D, D'Amico F et al. Paradoxical gastrointestinal effects of interleukin-17 blockers. *Ann Rheum Dis.* 2020 Sep;79(9):1132–8.

19. McGonagle D, Watad A, Sharif K et al. Why inhibition of IL-23 lacked efficacy in ankylosing spondylitis. *Front Immunol.* 2021 Mar 19;12:614255.

20. Sherlock JP, Joyce-Shaikh B, Turner SP et al. IL-23 induces spondyloarthropathy by acting on ROR-γt+CD3+CD4-CD8-entheseal resident T cells. *Nat Med.* 2012 Jul 1;18(7):1069–76.

21. Gelfand JM, Neimann AL, Shin DB et al. Risk of myocardial infarction in patients with psoriasis. *JAMA.* 2006 Oct 11;296(14):1735–41.

22. Takeshita J, Grewal S, Langan SM et al. Psoriasis and comorbid diseases: Epidemiology. *J Am Acad Dermatol.* 2017 Mar;76(3):377–90.

23. Dauden E, Blasco AJ, Bonanad C et al. Position statement for the management of comorbidities in psoriasis. *J Eur Acad Dermatol Venereol.* 2018 Dec;32(12):2058–73.

24. Ogdie A, Grewal SK, Noe MH et al. Risk of incident liver disease in patients with psoriasis, psoriatic arthritis, and rheumatoid arthritis: A population-based study. *J Invest Dermatol.* 2018 Apr;138(4):760–7.

25. Gelfand JM, Wan J, Zhang H et al. Risk of liver disease in patients with psoriasis, psoriatic arthritis, and rheumatoid arthritis receiving methotrexate: A population-based study. *J Am Acad Dermatol.* 2021 Jun;84(6):1636–43. Erratum in: *J Am Acad Dermatol.* 2023 Jul 20.

26. Ruan Z, Lu T, Chen Y et al. Association between psoriasis and nonalcoholic fatty liver disease among outpatient US adults. *JAMA Dermatol.* 2022 Jul 1;158(7):745–53.

27. Zheng Y, Danilenko DM, Valdez P et al. Interleukin-22, a T(H)17 cytokine, mediates IL-23-induced dermal inflammation and acanthosis. *Nature.* 2007 Feb 8;445(7128):648–51.

28. Akash MSH, Rehman K, Liaqat A. Tumor necrosis factor-alpha: Role in development of insulin resistance and pathogenesis of type 2 diabetes mellitus. *J Cell Biochem.* 2018 Jan;119(1):105–10.

29. Klingberg E, Björkman S, Eliasson B et al. Weight loss is associated with sustained improvement of disease activity and cardiovascular risk factors in patients with psoriatic arthritis and obesity: A prospective intervention study with two years of follow-up. *Arthritis Res Ther.* 2020 Oct 22;22(1):254.

30. Landgren AJ, Jonsson CA, Bilberg A et al. Serum IL-23 significantly decreased in obese patients with psoriatic arthritis six months after a structured weight loss intervention. *Arthritis Res Ther.* 2023 Jul 27;25(1):131.

5

Enteric Arthritis

SMARIKA SAPKOTA, YAWEN REN, AND KRISTINE A. KUHN

INFLAMMATORY BOWEL DISEASE

Introduction

Inflammatory bowel disease (IBD)–associated arthritis is an extraintestinal rheumatic manifestation of Crohn's disease (CD) or ulcerative colitis (UC) classified as a form of spondyloarthritis (SpA). Potentially, IBD and SpA fall along the same spectrum of disease. For example, SpA can be a preceding symptom in IBD, and asymptomatic bowel inflammation can be often found in patients with SpA (1). Genetically, the high frequency of HLA-B27 and other common alleles among the two disease states suggests shared mechanistic pathways. Management can be rendered more challenging when extraintestinal manifestations need to be considered in therapy selection. In this section, we will discuss the clinical characteristics of IBD-associated SpA, its proposed pathogenic pathways, and management recommendations.

Epidemiology

In North America, around 1 million to 2 million people are affected by IBD, with an incidence of 2.2 to 14.6 cases per 100,000 person-years (2). Within this population, arthritis has been described in up to 53% (3). More specifically, pooled prevalence for sacroiliitis, ankylosing spondylitis, and peripheral arthritis were 10%, 3%, and 13%, respectively. Males and females are affected equally (4, 5).

Pathophysiology

The precise pathway of gut inflammation leading to a systemic inflammatory response and inflammatory arthritis has yet to be established. Proposed mechanisms suggest that the increased gut barrier permeability during IBD provides microbes direct access to local tissues, subsequently stimulating an inflammatory response. Normally, the gut mucosal barrier keeps gut microbes away from the deeper lamina propria layer containing antigen presenting cells such as macrophages, dendritic cells, and lymphocytes. Once injury to the layer occurs, exposed microbes drive local Th17 cell–mediated inflammation (6). Th17 cells are a subgroup of T-helper cells, which are key players in the inflammatory response. Th17 cells have also been found in synovial fluid of patients with SpA and are positively correlated with systemic inflammation (7). Local inflammatory cytokines such as IL-23 drive production of IL-17, IL-22, and TNF from Th17 cells (1). IL-17 has several proinflammatory effects, and studies have shown that the IL-23/IL-17 pathway is an important driver of tissue damage in both IBD and SpA (7). An alternative hypothesis is the translocation of inflammatory cells such as macrophages, innate lymphocytes, and T cells from the gut to the joint to stimulate local inflammation in the enthesis, the pathogenic site for SpA (8).

The composition of microbial flora in the gut may also play a role in the development of SpA. Studies using HLA-B27 transgenic rat models have shown that microbe-free environments result

DOI: 10.1201/9781003367307-5

in the absence of the expected intestinal inflammation and arthritis (9). Fecal transfer of stool samples from mice with spontaneous ileitis into microbe-free mice prone to developing IBD results in the development of intestinal inflammation and arthritis. This effect was not observed when the samples were obtained from control mice (9). Although this indicates the microbiome is key to the evolution of disease, no single organism has been identified as the trigger for pathogenesis.

Genetic Predisposition

Genetic factors can affect responses of the adaptive and innate immune pathways. Polymorphisms in genes such as IL-23R, STAT3, and IL-12B, related to the IL-23/IL-17 pathway, have been described in CD, ankylosing spondylitis, and psoriatic arthritis (8). In addition, the presence of human leukocyte antigen (HLA) alleles such as HLA-B27, HLA-B35, HLA-B44 in IBD patients increases the risk of developing SpA. Specifically, HLA-B27 is positive in 25% to 78% of patients with IBD and ankylosing spondylitis (1). The role of HLA-B27 in gut and joint inflammation is thought to be due to protein misfolding, which leads to a cascade of inflammatory cytokines activating the IL-23/IL-17 pathway. Newer research suggests that HLA-B27 can present antigen from bacterial and host proteins to which clonally expanded T cells in ankylosing spondylitis and uveitis cross-react (10). However, other known genetic factors predisposing to IBD such as NOD2/CARD15 mutation, which is associated with Crohn's disease, do not increase prevalence for inflammatory arthritis.

Clinical Features

Historically, arthritis from IBD was recognized as different from rheumatoid arthritis due to the lack of positive rheumatoid factor, asymmetrical joint involvement, absence of rheumatoid nodules, and presence of axial involvement. Joint involvement in IBD-associated SpA is often categorized as axial or peripheral. Peripheral joint involvement is further separated into type 1 and type 2 subgroups depending on its association with IBD disease activity.

Axial joint involvement in IBD-associated arthritis is similar to idiopathic ankylosing spondylitis and can present with inflammatory low back pain and sacroiliitis (often bilateral) and even progress to ankylosis of the spine. Axial involvement is more commonly seen in CD than UC. Generally, it has been observed that axial disease activity does not correlate with bowel inflammation, and in fact, resection of inflamed bowel has no effect on axial disease (11).

Type 1 peripheral SpA is pauciarticular (less than 5 joints) with asymmetric involvement, with short self-limited joint flares that usually correlate with flares of IBD. This type is also associated with other nonarticular extraintestinal manifestations: inflammatory eye disease, aphthous stomatitis, erythema nodosum, and pyoderma gangrenosum. Commonly, the joints of the lower extremities are favored such as knees and ankles. Some studies have reported cases in which resection of the colon in patients UC had a curative effect on type 1 peripheral arthritis. Genetic associations include higher rates of HLA-B27, HLA-B35, and HLA-DRβ1*0103 (11, 12).

Type 2 peripheral arthritis lacks association with bowel disease flare. Involvement is often symmetrical, polyarticular (five or more joints), and chronic, lasting months to years. Common joints affected includes small joints such as MCPs. This type has a strong correlation with uveitis. Genetic associations include higher rates of HLA-B44 (11, 12).

Other clinical presentations include enthesitis and dactylitis. Enthesitis is the inflammation of the insertion sites of tendons and ligaments to the bone surface. Commonly, a patient can have inflammation involving the lateral and medial epicondyles, Achilles, or plantar fascia, causing pain on palpation of these insertion sites and often visible swelling on physical exam. Dactylitis is a diffuse tenosynovitis through an entire finger or toe, often called "sausage digit" due to resultant clinical appearance (11, 12).

Diagnostic Approach

Diagnosis is based on patient history, physical exam findings, and imaging. Laboratory tests play a smaller role compared to disorders like rheumatoid arthritis and connective tissue diseases. Symptoms that suggest inflammatory joint pain include joint swelling, morning stiffness, or pain that improves through the day with activity. Distribution of joint involvement and association with IBD disease activity are also helpful in diagnosis. Arthrocentesis of a swollen joint can provide information on whether the fluid is inflammatory and can help exclude other differential diagnoses such as crystalline disease or infection.

In axial disease, inflammatory back pain is classified as meeting four out of five criteria from Assessment of Spondylarthritis International Society (ASAS): age of onset < 40, insidious onset, improvement with exercise, no improvement with rest, pain at night (with improvement upon arising). Other criteria also include morning stiffness. These qualities help differentiate inflammatory pain from mechanical low back pain (13). Alternating buttock pain may indicate SI joint involvement. Hip pain can also occur and often be described by the patient as groin pain or pain referring to the medial thighs.

Physical exam findings, especially in those with advanced axial disease, could have reduced spinal mobility and range of motion. Objective measurements of joint mobility include Schober's test (measuring lumbar flexion distance at the level of L5), occiput-to-wall (measuring cervical neck extension), lateral spine side flexion, thoracic chest expansion, and hip internal rotation. These measurements are used to track the progression of axial disease in ankylosing spondylitis.

Radiographically, peripheral joints may not always reveal abnormalities, but occasionally, findings such as erosions, soft tissue swelling, and periostitis can be seen. In axial disease, radiographic evidence of sacroiliitis is more often bilateral and can range from sclerosis and erosions to complete joint fusion. The lower one-third of the SI joint is the synovial portion and most often affected due to inflammation of the adjacent subchondral bone. Radiographs of the spine can show vertebral body squaring with small erosions at the vertebral body corners, syndesmophytes, and ossification of the spinal ligaments that look like "whiskering" at the attachment sites. MRI of the pelvis should be performed to evaluate the SI joints in patients with normal radiographs but high suspicion for axial disease.

Elevations in CRP can help support diagnosis of IBD-associated SpA, but it can also be high in active bowel disease. The role of fecal calprotectin in evaluation of joint disease has yet to be determined (1). Studies have shown mixed results in terms of its association with joint disease activity and progression.

Management

Treatment of IBD-related arthritis requires active collaboration between the gastroenterologist and rheumatologist.

NSAIDs are traditionally used in idiopathic SpA as first-line therapy. However, in some studies, NSAIDs have been associated with IBD relapse due to reduced prostaglandins from COX-1/COX-2 inhibition. However, the data over NSAIDs causing IBD exacerbation is mixed. One meta-analysis study showed no correlation between NSAID use and IBD relapses (14). Overall, NSAIDs generally can be tried with a short course in those with quiet bowel disease.

Gluococorticoids are useful for bowel disease activity and peripheral arthritis. They have little effect on axial disease. Intra-articular glucocorticoid injections can also be considered when the arthritis is localized to a few peripheral joints to limit side effects of systemic steroids.

Traditional disease-modifying antirheumatic drugs (DMARDs) such as methotrexate, sulfasalazine, and leflunomide can be helpful in treating peripheral SpA but are not useful in prevention of disease progression in axial arthritis. In terms of bowel disease, methotrexate is effective as maintenance therapy in CD, and sulfasalazine has evidence supporting use in UC.

TNF inhibitors (TNFi; infliximab, etanercept, adalimumab, golimumab, certolizumab) are a mainstay in treating IBD-associated SpA because of their effectiveness in both axial and peripheral disease as well as IBD. TNFi have proven benefit preventing radiographic progression in psoriatic arthritis and ankylosing spondylitis (11, 12, 15). Among the different types of TNFi, infliximab and adalimumab are best studied in IBD with effectiveness in both CD and UC (16). Etanercept is less effective in IBD and uveitis, and may provoke increased flares of the latter (17). Screening for latent TB and viral hepatitis should be done prior to initiating TNFi therapy due to risk of reactivation.

IL-17 and IL-23 targeted therapies have been studied in IBD and SpA separately, and data are extrapolated for use in IBD-associated SpA. Ustekinumab is a monoclonal antibody against both IL-12/IL-23 with benefit shown in CD, UC, and psoriatic arthritis, but has minimal effect in axial disease (18). Secukinumab and ixekizumab are monoclonal antibodies targeting IL-17A and have demonstrated efficacy in psoriatic arthritis and ankylosing spondylitis. However, the clinical trial using secukinumab for CD resulted in increased disease activity compared to placebo (19). Therefore, IL-17A inhibitors are avoided in treatment of IBD. Interestingly, targeted IL-23 inhibition through blockage of the p19 subunit (guselkumab, tildrakizumab, and risankizumab) is effective in treatment of IBD and psoriatic arthritis, suggesting that it may be useful in IBD-associated peripheral SpA. However, similar to ustekinumab, IL-23 inhibition failed to treat ankylosing spondylitis (20, 21).

Vedolizumab, an inhibitor of α4β7 integrin whose receptor is MadCAM expressed on intestinal endothelial cells to mediate leukocyte migration into the intestine, is an effective therapy for UC. However, case reports have described flares of SpA in patients with IBD on this therapy. It is unclear whether blockade of leukocyte trafficking to the gut caused them to migrate to the joints and stimulate inflammation or if the gut-specific therapy unmasked previously partially treated SpA (22).

Other biologics with limited data include JAK inhibitors (baricitinib, tofacitinib, upadacitinib), which are approved for patients with IBD, although there is variance in efficacy and approval for UC versus CD between members of the class (23). JAK inhibitors are also effective for psoriatic arthritis and ankylosing spondylitis, suggesting that they may be effective in IBD-associated SpA (24).

CELIAC DISEASE

Introduction

Celiac disease is a systemic immune-mediated disease incited by dietary gluten in genetically susceptible individuals. Gluten is a protein complex which is found in wheat, rye, and barley. This is an autoimmune condition characterized by a broad range of clinical presentations with variable damage to small-intestinal mucosa (25).

Epidemiology

The worldwide prevalence of celiac disease (CeD) is 0.6% to 1.0% with wide regional differences partly because it is often underrecognized (26, 27). In one study, only 21% of those who screened positive for laboratory testing had been clinically recognized (28). The prevalence is 1.5 to 2 times higher among women compared to men and is increased among persons with affected first-degree relatives (10% to 15%), IgA deficiency (9%), or other autoimmune diseases such as type 1 diabetes (3% to 16%) and Hashimoto's thyroiditis (5%). Down's and Turner's syndromes also have increased prevalence of CeD (5% and 3%, respectively) (29–33).

Pathophysiology

Gluten is a heterogeneous molecule from which digested fractions are a mixture of peptides rich in glutamine and proline residues called gliadins. Gliadin peptides are a substrate for tissue transglutaminase that converts the glutamine into negatively charged glutamate residues (a process called deamination), which makes the deaminated gliadin peptides suitable for interaction with MHC class II (34). The presentation of gliadin peptides by MHC class II molecules to CD4 + T cell leads to the activation of humoral responses with lymphocyte infiltration in the lamina propria with dominance of CD4+ T cells and plasma cells targeting gliadin (35, 36). Patients with CeD also develop autoantibodies against tissue transglutaminase, which suggests that CeD has an autoimmune component despite its induction by dietary antigen (37, 38).

Ultimately, inflammation of the small intestine causes derangement in the architecture of the mucosa, with flattening of the villi, infiltration of lymphocytes in the epithelium, and increased density and depth of the crypts. These changes occur in a continuum from normal to complete flattening of the villi in a slow progression (39).

Genetic Predisposition

About 90% of patients with CeD carry major histocompatibility (MHC) class II molecules of the HLA-DQ2 haplotype (DQA1*0501/DQB1*0201), compared to one-third of the general population carrying this haplotype. Within the remaining 10% of patients with CeD, 5% have HLA-DQ8 haplotype (DQA1*0301/DQB1*0302), and the remaining 5% of the patients with celiac disease has one of the other DQ2 haplotypes DQB1*0201 or DQA1*0501 (40).

Clinical Features

Symptoms of CeD include fatigue, weight loss, oral ulcers, abdominal discomfort, and chronic diarrhea, but these are experienced in only 40% to 50% of patients (25). Additional features include iron deficiency anemia, low bone mineral density, and a condition called dermatitis herpetiformis, an intensely pruritic vesicular rash whose pathology reveals IgA deposition on immunofluorescence (41). Arthralgia and arthritis can occur in ~20% of patients with CeD. The arthritis is seronegative and oligoarticular, with some patients experiencing enthesitis or exhibiting sacroiliitis on imaging (42–44). Often, CeD can be seen in conjunction with other autoimmune diseases such as type 1 diabetes, autoimmune thyroid disease, Sjogren's syndrome, and autoimmune hepatitis, among others (25, 45, 46). Rarely, T cell lymphoma and adenocarcinoma of the jejunum are complications of celiac disease, more typically in patients with history of suboptimal disease control (47).

Table 5.1 Extraintestinal Manifestations of Celiac Disease

Category	Manifestation
Neurologic	Peripheral neuropathy
	Headache
	Depression/anxiety
	Cerebellar ataxia
	Epilepsy
Endocrine	Type 1 diabetes
	Autoimmune thyroid disease
	Addison's disease
Cardiac	Idiopathic dilated cardiomyopathy
	Autoimmune myocarditis
Hepatic	Primary biliary cirrhosis
	Autoimmune hepatitis
	Autoimmune cholangitis
Rheumatologic	Oligoarticular arthritis
	Juvenile arthritis
	Sjogren's syndrome
	Sarcoidosis
Other	Anemia
	Osteoporosis
	Pancreatitis
	Alopecia areata

Adapted from Hernandez et al. (48)

Table 5.1 provides a summary of various disease associations and extraintestinal manifestations of celiac disease.

Diagnosis

Serologic testing for IgA autoantibodies against tissue transglutaminase is usually sufficient to establish a diagnosis of CeD. In the setting of a borderline positive result, IgA antiendomysial antibodies can be used as a confirmatory test. As IgA deficiency increases the risk for CeD and can confound testing, it is recommended that IgA levels also be tested to exclude this as a cause for a negative result. IgG antibodies to deaminated gliadin can be used in the setting of IgA deficiency. Table 5.2 summarizes the sensitivity and specificity of antibody testing for CeD. However, the sensitivity of serologic testing is markedly reduced in patients with a gluten-restricted diet. Testing for HLA-DQ2 and HLA-DQ8 may be useful as they have a high negative predictive value (49–51).

A biopsy of the small intestine is confirmatory in patients with suspected CeD. Pathognomonic characteristics include increases in the number of intraepithelial lymphocytes, crypt hypertrophy, and villous atrophy (25).

Treatment

The gold standard treatment is a gluten-free diet with no wheat, rye, or barley proteins. Maintenance of a gluten-free diet leads to resolution of symptoms and intestinal healing within 6 to 24 months (25).

Table 5.2 Sensitivity and Specificity of Testing for CeD

Test	Sensitivity (Range)	Specificity (Range)
IgA anti TTG antibodies	> 95 (74–100)	> 95 (78–100)
IgA antiendomysial antibodies	> 90 (83–100)	98 (95–100)
IgG deaminated gliadin peptides	> 90 (80–99)	> 90 (86–97)
HLA-DQ2 or HLA-DQ8	91 (83–97)	54 (12–68)

WHIPPLE'S DISEASE

Introduction

Whipple's disease (WD) is a rare, systemic infectious illness caused by the bacterium *Tropheryma whipplei* often characterized by weight loss, diarrhea, and arthralgia (52, 53). This disease was fatal until the introduction of antibiotics in 1952 (54). The aim of this section is to focus on rheumatologic manifestations of this heterogeneous disease as well as to highlight some of the key concepts related to pathogenesis, diagnosis, and treatment of WD.

Epidemiology

The approximate incidence is less than 1 per 1,000,000 and predominantly affects middle-aged white men of European ancestry (~89% of cases) with mean age of 49 years. *T. whipplei* has been identified in sewers and human stool, thought to be spread by oral–oral and fecal–oral transmission (55).

Genetics and Pathogenesis

Chronic systemic infection with *T. whipplei* seems only to occur in predisposed individuals (10); however, asymptomatic carriage of *T. whipplei* is frequent, ranging up to one-third of some populations (56). Genetic associations include MHC class II alleles DRB1*13 and DQB1*06 and MHC class I B27 (57).

When infected with *T. whipplei*, many individuals will subsequently develop a protective immune response. However, those who develop Whipple's disease (WD) seem to lack an effective immune response. *T. whipplei* replicates within monocytes and macrophages, particularly within the duodenal mucosa, and is a hallmark of the disease. These monocytes and macrophages take on a regulatory phenotype characterized by high interleukin (IL)-10, IL-16, and chemokine ligand 18 (CCL18) production and decreased IL-12 and interferon (IFN)γ (58, 59). This leads to inefficient elimination of intracellular pathogen, lack of T helper cell responses, and reduced antibodies targeting *T. whipplei* (58–61). Hence, macrophages ingest *T. whipplei*, but due to impaired phagosomes and adaptive immune responses, the bacteria survive and spread through apoptosis of infected cells (62–64).

Clinical Features

WD is characterized by two stages—a prodromal stage and a much later steady-state stage, with the average duration between them around 6 years. In cases of patients receiving immunosuppressive therapy, a more rapid clinical progression could occur. The prodromal stage comprises nonspecific findings, mainly arthralgia and arthritis. The steady-state stage is characterized by weight loss, diarrhea, and other various manifestations including neurologic, cardiac, ophthalmic, pulmonary, or hematologic (65).

Joint involvement has been reported in 65% to 90% of patients with classic WD. Intermittent migratory arthralgia as well as polyarticular > oligoarticular arthritis are common features. Typically, the polyarthritis is a seronegative, nondestructive joint disease affecting small peripheral joints with migratory characteristics (66–68). Arthralgia precedes definite diagnosis of WD by a mean 6 to 7 years and often improves spontaneously once diarrheal symptoms occur (67). Less frequently in WD, a chronic seronegative, erosive polyarthritis has also been described (66).

Features of classic WD are outlined in Table 5.3.

Diagnosis

The gold standard test for WD is the identification of *T. whipplei* in small bowel biopsy. Traditionally, PAS staining is performed on the biopsy tissue, which will identify magenta-stained inclusions within macrophages. This alone is not sufficient for diagnosis. A confirmatory PCR for the *T. whipplei* bacterium is performed on the tissue. A similar approach can be used for other tissues such as synovial fluid and CSF in which *T. whipplei* is suspected to be present (55, 67).

Treatment

Antibiotics that can cross the blood–brain barrier, such as trimethoprim-sulfamethoxazole, are favored over more traditional therapies such as tetracycline, which has a relapse rate of 28% following treatment. The recommended treatment is oral administration of 160 mg of trimethoprim and 800

Table 5.3 Frequency of Symptoms in WD

Feature	Prevalence
Weight loss	90%
Arthralgia/Arthritis	85%
Diarrhea	75%
Abdominal pain	60%
Fever	45%
Lymphadenopathy	45%
Hyperpigmentation	35%
Hypotension	35%
Peripheral edema	30%
Occult blood loss	25%
Myalgia	25%
Neurologic involvement (ophthalmoplegia, myoclonus, seizures, ataxia, cognitive change)	15%
Chronic cough	15%
Splenomegaly	15%
Hepatomegaly	10%
Ascites	10%

Adapted from Marth et al. (67).

mg of sulfamethoxazole twice per day for 1 to 2 years, usually preceded by parenteral administration of streptomycin (1 gm per day) together with penicillin G (1.2 million U per day) or ceftriaxone (2 gm daily) for 2 weeks. However, it is still possible to have recurrence with this strategy (55, 67).

Prognosis

With targeted treatment with antibiotics that cross the blood–brain barrier, proof of eradication of *T. whipplei*, remission can be achieved. However, lifelong clinical follow-up is advised since relapses can still occur after many years. Untreated WD is fatal, but the exact mortality rate of treated WD is not known. Relapses are common and responsible for disease morbidity and mortality. Historically reported relapse rates are around 30%. Relapses commonly occur early after the cessation of antibiotics but even can occur after many years in patients in clinical remission and without treatment (55, 67). Late relapses of CNS disease can occur and might have a progressive or detrimental course. A quarter of patients with CNS infection die within 4 years, whereas another quarter develop debilitating sequelae (69).

CLOSTRIDIOIDES DIFFICILE–ASSOCIATED REACTIVE ARTHRITIS

Introduction

Clostridioides difficile infection (CDI) is a toxin-mediated intestinal disease caused by spore-forming anaerobic, gram-positive bacilli. Aside from its well-known gastrointestinal manifestations, CDI has also been known to cause reactive arthritis. Information on reactive arthritis associated with CDI is mainly derived from case series and reports in adults (70–75).

Epidemiology

Between 2011 and 2017, there was a decline in the incidence of CDI in the United States (from 154.9 to 143.6 per 100,000 persons), primarily driven by a decrease in healthcare–associated infections (8). In Europe, the incidence of healthcare-associated CDI is 4.2 per 10,000 patient-days, with a case-fatality rate of 9% within 3 months after diagnosis (76).

Pathogenesis

Antibiotic use has been the major risk factor for CDI. Two major roles for antibiotics in the pathogenesis of CDI have been (1) the disruption of barrier function by the normal colonic microbiota, providing a niche for *C. difficile* to multiply, and (2) development of *C. difficile* resistance to clindamycin and fluoroquinolones appears to select strains with increased virulence. Other risk factors include advanced age and comorbidities such as cirrhosis, heart disease, pulmonary disease, hemodialysis, and immunocompromised status (76–82).

In addition to the known gastrointestinal manifestations of CDI, there have been reports of extracolonic manifestation including bacteremia, cellulitis, pancreatic or splenic abscesses, pleural empyema, osteomyelitis, native or artificial joint infections, and appendicitis (76–82).

Reactive arthritis (ReA) may also occur, although the exact prevalence of this complication is not known (71–75). One hypothesis proposes that immunologic tolerance is interrupted during *C. difficile* antigenic presentation. Although ReA due to other enteric pathogens such as *Salmonella* or *Chlamydia trachomatis* is characterized by circulating bacterial lipopolysaccharide (LPS) prior to the onset of ReA, CD is devoid of LPS (83). Rather, *C. difficile* toxin A, which increases epithelial permeability of the intestinal barrier, may allow passage of other bacterial antigens or LPS to the circulation (20). Passage of such bacterial products could result in a cascade of immune activation that ultimately targets joint tissues in susceptible patients (84).

HLA B27 may have a role in CDI-associated ReA (84). One case series identified a higher prevalence of HLA B27 in patients who developed CDI-associated ReA; those without an HLA B27 genotype were able to resolve the arthritis without antibiotic treatment, suggesting that there is a sterile inflammation occurring within the joint rather than bacterial translocation to that site (84, 85). Inflammatory mediators such as calprotectin (product of neutrophil activation), IL-8, or IL-23 have been identified in the synovial fluid and circulation of patients with CDI-associated ReA, demonstrating pathogenic similarities to IBD-associated SpA (86–88).

Clinical Features

ReA occurred at a median 10 days after CDI with an initial presentation of oligoarthritis (44%), polyarthritis (38%), or monoarthritis (18%). The most commonly involved joints were ankles (63.6%) and knees (59.1%). Episodes of ReA lasted from 5 to 800 days with median of 42 days. About 90% of cases spontaneously resolved, and 55% of patients required use of nonsteroidal anti-inflammatory drugs (84).

Diagnosis

Diagnosis of CDI-associated ReA is based upon:

1. Evidence of aseptic synovitis that developed during or immediately after diarrhea and/or colitis;
2. Diarrhea appearing after a course of systemic antimicrobial therapy;
3. Microbiologic proof of CDI (either positive stool culture or assay for toxin); and
4. Absence of other causes of colitis and arthritis (89).

Treatment

Treatment of CDI with either oral vancomycin or metronidazole leads to resolution of both the colitis and ReA in most cases. In addition, NSAIDs, intra-articular steroids, or oral steroids may be necessary for the treatment of ReA (71, 75, 84, 89, 90).

CONCLUSIONS

Noninfectious and infectious intestinal pathologies have strong connections with inflammation in the joints. A common underlying pathophysiology connecting the gut to the joint is mucosal immune cell development in the intestine that influences systemic immune functions. For most of these conditions, a thorough history and physical exam should guide the necessary radiologic and laboratory tests to confirm a diagnosis. When the underlying cause is infectious, often, antibiotic therapy is sufficient to treat the arthritis. However, when the cause is sterile inflammation, as in the case of IBD, a combination of disease-modifying agents, usually biologics, is required for the treatment of arthritis.

REFERENCES

1. Fragoulis GE, Liava C, Daoussis D et al. Inflammatory bowel diseases and spondyloarthropathies: From pathogenesis to treatment. *World J Gastroenterol.* 2019;25(18):2162–76.
2. Loftus EV, Jr. Clinical epidemiology of inflammatory bowel disease: Incidence, prevalence, and environmental influences. *Gastroenterol.* 2004;126(6):1504–17.
3. Wollheim FA. Enteropathic arthritis: How do the joints talk with the gut? *Curr Opin Rheumatol.* 2001;13(4):305–9.
4. Karreman MC, Luime JJ, Hazes JMW et al. The prevalence and incidence of axial and peripheral spondyloarthritis in inflammatory bowel disease: A systematic review and meta-analysis. *J Crohns Colitis.* 2017;11(5):631–42.
5. Gravallese EM, Kantrowitz FG. Arthritic manifestations of inflammatory bowel disease. *Am J Gastroenterol.* 1988;83(7):703–9.
6. Ashrafi M, Kuhn KA, Weisman MH. The arthritis connection to Inflammatory Bowel Disease (IBD): Why has it taken so long to understand it? *RMD Open.* 2021;7(1).
7. Zizzo G, De Santis M, Bosello SL et al. Synovial fluid-derived T helper 17 cells correlate with inflammatory activity in arthritis,

irrespectively of diagnosis. *Clin Immunol.* 2011;138(1):107–16.

8. Lefferts AR, Norman E, Claypool DJ et al. Cytokine competent gut-joint migratory T cells contribute to inflammation in the joint. *Front Immunol.* 2022;13:932393.

9. Taurog JD, Richardson JA, Croft JT et al. The germfree state prevents development of gut and joint inflammatory disease in HLA-B27 transgenic rats. *J Exp Med.* 1994;180(6):2359–64.

10. Yang X, Garner LI, Zvyagin IV et al. Autoimmunity-associated T cell receptors recognize HLA-B*27-bound peptides. *Nature.* 2022;612(7941):771–7.

11. Peluso R, Di Minno MN, Iervolino S et al. Enteropathic spondyloarthritis: From diagnosis to treatment. *Clin Dev Immunol.* 2013;2013:631408.

12. Ono K, Kishimoto M, Deshpande GA et al. Clinical characteristics of patients with spondyloarthritis and inflammatory bowel disease versus inflammatory bowel disease-related arthritis. *Rheumatol Int.* 2022;42(10):1751–66.

13. Rudwaleit M, Landewe R, van der Heijde D et al. The development of Assessment of SpondyloArthritis International Society classification criteria for axial spondyloarthritis (part I): Classification of paper patients by expert opinion including uncertainty appraisal. *Ann Rheum Dis.* 2009;68(6):770–6.

14. Moninuola OO, Milligan W, Lochhead P et al. Systematic review with meta-analysis: Association between acetaminophen and Nonsteroidal Anti-Inflammatory Drugs (NSAIDs) and risk of Crohn's disease and ulcerative colitis exacerbation. *Aliment Pharmacol Ther.* 2018;47(11):1428–39.

15. Soriano ER, McHugh NJ. Therapies for peripheral joint disease in psoriatic arthritis: A systematic review. *J Rheumatol.* 2006;33(7):1422–30.

16. Pouillon L, Bossuyt P, Vanderstukken J et al. Management of patients with inflammatory bowel disease and spondyloarthritis. *Expert Rev Clin Pharmacol.* 2017;10(12):1363–74.

17. Guillot X, Prati C, Sondag M et al. Etanercept for treating axial spondyloarthritis. *Expert Opin Biol Ther.* 2017;17(9):1173–81.

18. Deodhar A, Gensler LS, Sieper J et al. Three multicenter, randomized, double-blind, placebo-controlled studies evaluating the efficacy and safety of ustekinumab in axial spondyloarthritis. *Arthritis Rheumatol.* 2019;71(2):258–70.

19. Hueber W, Sands BE, Lewitzky S et al. Secukinumab, a human anti-IL-17A monoclonal antibody, for moderate to severe Crohn's disease: Unexpected results of a randomised, double-blind placebo-controlled trial. *Gut.* 2012;61(12):1693–700.

20. McDonald BD, Dyer EC, Rubin DT. IL-23 monoclonal antibodies for IBD: So many, so different? *J Crohns Colitis.* 2022;16(Suppl 2):ii42–53.

21. Braun J, Landewe RB. No efficacy of anti-IL-23 therapy for axial spondyloarthritis in randomised controlled trials but in post-hoc analyses of psoriatic arthritis-related "physician-reported spondylitis"? *Ann Rheum Dis.* 2022;81(4):466–8.

22. Dubash S, Marianayagam T, Tinazzi I et al. Emergence of severe spondyloarthropathy-related entheseal pathology following successful vedolizumab therapy for inflammatory bowel disease. *Rheumatol (Oxford).* 2019;58(6):963–8.

23. Herrera-deGuise C, Serra-Ruiz X, Lastiri E et al. JAK inhibitors: A new dawn for oral therapies in inflammatory bowel diseases. *Front Med (Lausanne).* 2023;10:1089099.

24. McInnes IB, Szekanecz Z, McGonagle D et al. A review of JAK-STAT signalling in the pathogenesis of spondyloarthritis and the role of JAK inhibition. *Rheumatol (Oxford).* 2022;61(5):1783–94.

25. Fasano A, Catassi C. Clinical practice: Celiac disease. *N Engl J Med.* 2012;367(25):2419–26.

26. Fasano A, Berti I, Gerarduzzi T et al. Prevalence of celiac disease in at-risk and not-at-risk groups in the United States: A large multicenter study. *Arch Intern Med.* 2003;163(3):286–92.

27. Biagi F, Klersy C, Balduzzi D et al. Are we not over-estimating the prevalence of coeliac disease in the general population? *Ann Med.* 2010;42(8):557–61.

28. Mustalahti K, Catassi C, Reunanen A et al. The prevalence of celiac disease in

Europe: Results of a centralized, international mass screening project. *Ann Med.* 2010;42(8):587–95.

29. Wouters J, Weijerman ME, van Furth AM et al. Prospective human leukocyte antigen, endomysium immunoglobulin A antibodies, and transglutaminase antibodies testing for celiac disease in children with down syndrome. *J Pediatr.* 2009;154(2):239–42.

30. Volta U, Tovoli F, Caio G. Clinical and immunological features of celiac disease in patients with Type 1 diabetes mellitus. *Expert Rev Gastroenterol Hepatol.* 2011;5(4):479–87.

31. Rubio-Tapia A, Van Dyke CT, Lahr BD et al. Predictors of family risk for celiac disease: A population-based study. *Clin Gastroenterol Hepatol.* 2008;6(9):983–7.

32. Lenhardt A, Plebani A, Marchetti F et al. Role of human-tissue transglutaminase IgG and anti-gliadin IgG antibodies in the diagnosis of coeliac disease in patients with selective immunoglobulin A deficiency. *Dig Liver Dis.* 2004;36(11):730–4.

33. Frost AR, Band MM, Conway GS. Serological screening for coeliac disease in adults with Turner's syndrome: Prevalence and clinical significance of endomysium antibody positivity. *Eur J Endocrinol.* 2009;160(4):675–9.

34. Hausch F, Shan L, Santiago NA et al. Intestinal digestive resistance of immunodominant gliadin peptides. *Am J Physiol Gastrointest Liver Physiol.* 2002;283(4):G996–1003.

35. van de Wal Y, Kooy Y, van Veelen P et al. Selective deamidation by tissue transglutaminase strongly enhances gliadin-specific T cell reactivity. *J Immunol.* 1998;161(4):1585–8.

36. Molberg O, McAdam SN, Korner R et al. Tissue transglutaminase selectively modifies gliadin peptides that are recognized by gut-derived T cells in celiac disease. *Nat Med.* 1998;4(6):713–17.

37. Dieterich W, Ehnis T, Bauer M et al. Identification of tissue transglutaminase as the autoantigen of celiac disease. *Nat Med.* 1997;3(7):797–801.

38. Baklien K, Brandtzaeg P, Fausa O. Immunoglobulins in jejunal mucosa and serum from patients with adult coeliac disease. *Scand J Gastroenterol.* 1977;12(2):149–59.

39. Marsh MN. Gluten, major histocompatibility complex, and the small intestine: A molecular and immunobiologic approach to the spectrum of gluten sensitivity ("celiac sprue"). *Gastroenterol.* 1992;102(1):330–54.

40. Karell K, Louka AS, Moodie SJ et al. HLA types in celiac disease patients not carrying the DQA1*05-DQB1*02 (DQ2) heterodimer: Results from the European Genetics Cluster on celiac disease. *Hum Immunol.* 2003;64(4):469–77.

41. Caproni M, Antiga E, Melani L et al. Guidelines for the diagnosis and treatment of dermatitis herpetiformis. *J Eur Acad Dermatol Venereol.* 2009;23(6):633–8.

42. Vereckei E, Mester A, Hodinka L et al. Back pain and sacroiliitis in long-standing adult celiac disease: A cross-sectional and follow-up study. *Rheumatol Int.* 2010;30(4):455–60.

43. Daron C, Soubrier M, Mathieu S. Occurrence of rheumatic symptoms in celiac disease: A meta-analysis: Comment on the article "Osteoarticular manifestations of celiac disease and non-celiac gluten hypersensitivity" by Dos Santos and Liote. *Joint Bone Spine.* 2016. https://doi.org/10.1016/j.jbspin.2016.09.007. *Joint Bone Spine.* 2017;84(5):645–6.

44. Bourne JT, Kumar P, Huskisson EC et al. Arthritis and coeliac disease. *Ann Rheum Dis.* 1985;44(9):592–8.

45. Talal AH, Murray JA, Goeken JA et al. Celiac disease in an adult population with insulin-dependent diabetes mellitus: Use of endomysial antibody testing. *Am J Gastroenterol.* 1997;92(8):1280–4.

46. Sattar N, Lazare F, Kacer M et al. Celiac disease in children, adolescents, and young adults with autoimmune thyroid disease. *J Pediatr.* 2011;158(2):272–5 e1.

47. Sharaiha RZ, Lebwohl B, Reimers L et al. Increasing incidence of enteropathy-associated T-cell lymphoma in the United States, 1973–2008. *Cancer.* 2012;118(15):3786–92.

48. Hernandez L, Green PH. Extraintestinal manifestations of celiac disease. *Curr Gastroenterol Rep.* 2006;8(5):383–9.

49. Zintzaras E, Germenis AE. Performance of antibodies against tissue transglutaminase for the diagnosis of celiac disease: Meta-analysis. *Clin Vaccine Immunol.* 2006;13(2):187–92.

50. Tonutti E, Visentini D, Picierno A et al. Diagnostic efficacy of the ELISA test for the detection of deamidated anti-gliadin peptide antibodies in the diagnosis and monitoring of celiac disease. *J Clin Lab Anal.* 2009;23(3):165–71.

51. Giersiepen K, Lelgemann M, Stuhldreher N et al. Accuracy of diagnostic antibody tests for coeliac disease in children: Summary of an evidence report. *J Pediatr Gastroenterol Nutr.* 2012;54(2):229–41.

52. Relman DA, Schmidt TM, MacDermott RP et al. Identification of the uncultured bacillus of Whipple's disease. *N Engl J Med.* 1992;327(5):293–301.

53. Obst W, von Arnim U, Malfertheiner P. Whipple's disease. *Viszeralmedizin.* 2014;30(3):167–72.

54. Copland SM, Colvin SH. Intestinal lipodystrophy or Whipple's disease. *Surgery.* 1949;26(4):688–98.

55. Fenollar F, Puechal X, Raoult D. Whipple's disease. *N Engl J Med.* 2007;356(1):55–66.

56. Fenollar F, Lagier JC, Raoult D. Tropheryma whipplei and Whipple's disease. *J Infect.* 2014;69(2):103–12.

57. Martinetti M, Biagi F, Badulli C et al. The HLA alleles DRB1*13 and DQB1*06 are associated to Whipple's disease. *Gastroenterol.* 2009;136(7):2289–94.

58. Moos V, Kunkel D, Marth T et al. Reduced peripheral and mucosal Tropheryma whipplei-specific Th1 response in patients with Whipple's disease. *J Immunol.* 2006;177(3):2015–22.

59. Marth T, Neurath M, Cuccherini BA et al. Defects of monocyte interleukin 12 production and humoral immunity in Whipple's disease. *Gastroenterol.* 1997;113(2):442–8.

60. Schinnerling K, Moos V, Geelhaar A et al. Regulatory T cells in patients with Whipple's disease. *J Immunol.* 2011;187(8):4061–7.

61. Marth T, Kleen N, Stallmach A et al. Dysregulated peripheral and mucosal Th1/Th2 response in Whipple's disease. *Gastroenterol.* 2002;123(5):1468–77.

62. Gorvel L, Al Moussawi K, Ghigo E et al. Tropheryma whipplei, the Whipple's disease bacillus, induces macrophage apoptosis through the extrinsic pathway. *Cell Death Dis.* 2010;1(4):e34.

63. Ghigo E, Barry AO, Pretat L et al. IL-16 promotes T. whipplei replication by inhibiting phagosome conversion and modulating macrophage activation. *PLoS One.* 2010;5(10):e13561.

64. Desnues B, Raoult D, Mege JL. IL-16 is critical for Tropheryma whipplei replication in Whipple's disease. *J Immunol.* 2005;175(7):4575–82.

65. Wilson KH, Blitchington R, Frothingham R et al. Phylogeny of the Whipple's-disease-associated bacterium. *Lancet.* 1991;338(8765):474–5.

66. Puechal X. Whipple disease and arthritis. *Curr Opin Rheumatol.* 2001;13(1):74–9.

67. Marth T, Moos V, Muller C et al. Tropheryma whipplei infection and Whipple's disease. *Lancet Infect Dis.* 2016;16(3):e13–22.

68. Durand DV, Lecomte C, Cathebras P et al. Whipple disease: Clinical review of 52 cases: The SNFMI Research Group on Whipple disease: Societe Nationale Francaise de Medecine Interne. *Med (Baltimore).* 1997;76(3):170–84.

69. Panegyres PK. Diagnosis and management of Whipple's disease of the brain. *Pract Neurol.* 2008;8(5):311–17.

70. Rupnik M, Wilcox MH, Gerding DN. Clostridium difficile infection: New developments in epidemiology and pathogenesis. *Nat Rev Microbiol.* 2009;7(7):526–36.

71. Birnbaum J, Bartlett JG, Gelber AC. Clostridium difficile: An under-recognized cause of reactive arthritis? *Clin Rheumatol.* 2008;27(2):253–5.

72. Hayward RS, Wensel RH, Kibsey P. Relapsing Clostridium difficile colitis and Reiter's syndrome. *Am J Gastroenterol.* 1990;85(6):752–6.

73. Jacobs A, Barnard K, Fishel R et al. Extracolonic manifestations of Clostridium difficile infections: Presentation of 2 cases and review of the literature. *Med (Baltimore).* 2001;80(2):88–101.

74. Prati C, Bertolini E, Toussirot E et al. Reactive arthritis due to Clostridium difficile. *Joint Bone Spine.* 2010;77(2):190–2.

75. Kocar IH, Caliskaner Z, Pay S et al. Clostridium difficile infection in patients with reactive arthritis of undetermined etiology. *Scand J Rheumatol*. 1998;27(5):357–62.

76. Bauer MP, Notermans DW, van Benthem BH et al. Clostridium difficile infection in Europe: A hospital-based survey. *Lancet*. 2011;377(9759):63–73.

77. Riley TV, Karthigasu KT. Chronic osteomyelitis due to Clostridium difficile. *Br Med J* (Clin Res Ed). 1982;284(6324):1217–18.

78. Sofianou DC. Pancreatic abscess caused by Clostridium difficile. *Eur J Clin Microbiol Infect Dis*. 1988;7(4):528–9.

79. Simpson AJ, Das SS, Tabaqchali S. Nosocomial empyema caused by Clostridium difficile. *J Clin Pathol*. 1996;49(2):172–3.

80. Kumar N, Flanagan P, Wise C et al. Splenic abscess caused by Clostridium difficile. *Eur J Clin Microbiol Infect Dis*. 1997;16(12):938–9.

81. Bhargava A, Sen P, Swaminathan A et al. Rapidly progressive necrotizing fasciitis and gangrene due to Clostridium difficile: Case report. *Clin Infect Dis*. 2000;30(6):954–5.

82. Libby DB, Bearman G. Bacteremia due to Clostridium difficile—Review of the literature. *Int J Infect Dis*. 2009;13(5):e305–9.

83. Granfors K, Jalkanen S, Lindberg AA et al. Salmonella lipopolysaccharide in synovial cells from patients with reactive arthritis. *Lancet*. 1990;335(8691):685–8.

84. Legendre P, Lalande V, Eckert C et al. Clostridium difficile associated reactive arthritis: Case report and literature review. *Anaerobe*. 2016;38:76–80.

85. Ben Abdelghani K, Gerard-Dran D, Morel J et al. Clostridium difficile associated reactive arthritis. *Rev Med Interne*. 2010;31(3):e13–15.

86. Bressler B, Panaccione R, Fedorak RN et al. Clinicians' guide to the use of fecal calprotectin to identify and monitor disease activity in inflammatory bowel disease. *Can J Gastroenterol Hepatol*. 2015;29(7):369–72.

87. Konikoff MR, Denson LA. Role of fecal calprotectin as a biomarker of intestinal inflammation in inflammatory bowel disease. *Inflamm Bowel Dis*. 2006;12(6):524–34.

88. Hammer HB, Kvien TK, Glennas A et al. A longitudinal study of calprotectin as an inflammatory marker in patients with reactive arthritis. *Clin Exp Rheumatol*. 1995;13(1):59–64.

89. Putterman C, Rubinow A. Reactive arthritis associated with Clostridium difficile pseudomembranous colitis. *Semin Arthritis Rheum*. 1993;22(6):420–6.

90. Horton DB, Strom BL, Putt ME et al. Epidemiology of clostridium difficile infection-associated reactive arthritis in children: An underdiagnosed, potentially morbid condition. *JAMA Pediatr*. 2016;170(7):e160217.

6

Systemic Lupus Erythematosus

MICHAEL MACKLIN AND KIMBERLY TROTTER

INTRODUCTION

Systemic lupus erythematosus (SLE) is a complex, multiorgan, autoimmune disease with an incredibly wide range of clinical presentations. In the United States, SLE has an incidence and prevalence of about 46.9 and 366.6 cases per 100,000 person-years, respectively, as of 2016 (1). Significant ethnic disparities exist within the United States: African American, American Indian, and Alaska Native populations exhibit more than double the incidence and prevalence of SLE compared with white populations (1). African American patients are also more commonly afflicted by lupus nephritis, along with American Indian SLE patients demonstrating significantly higher mortality compared with other populations. Mortality in hospital is heavily weighted toward infections, followed by cardiac causes (1).

SLE requires expert opinion for diagnosis, though criteria for standardization of patients for research purposes do exist, which can help act as a screening framework for manifestations of the disease. For SLE, the most recent classification criteria are the 2019 EULAR/ACR criteria (2). In these criteria, all patients must have a positive ANA, followed by obtaining 10 or more points based on involved domains. These domains include constitutional, hematologic, neuropsychiatric, mucocutaneous, serosal, musculoskeletal, renal, presence of low complement proteins, presence of antiphospholipid antibodies, and presence of SLE-specific antibodies. It is important to note that these criteria do not capture many lupus manifestations and that patients may be diagnosed with SLE despite not meeting these criteria in clinical practice.

Treatment of SLE is complex and individualized. Various doses of corticosteroids may be used to induce remission, although their long-term risks remain a concern and necessitate early introduction of additional agents. Hydroxychloroquine is uniquely considered as anchor therapy in all SLE patients unless contraindications exist given its success at reducing flares with an overall excellent safety profile. The conventional DMARDs mycophenolate, methotrexate, and azathioprine can be used for improving disease control, with mycophenolate offering particular utility for lupus nephritis. Cyclophosphamide remains an option for life-threatening or refractory disease, with rituximab reserved for hematological complications (3). Belimumab, a newer monoclonal antibody targeting B-Lymphocyte stimulator, can be used in a variety of manifestations including class III/IV nephritis (3, 4). Voclosporin, a recently approved calcineurin inhibitor, is approved for lupus nephritis including class III/IV/V as an add-on therapy (5). Anifrolumab, an anti-type 1 interferon receptor antibody, has a niche in severe SLE-driven skin manifestations (6).

This chapter will closely examine the clinical manifestations as well as explore the diagnosis/treatment of gastrointestinal disease in SLE.

DOI: 10.1201/9781003367307-6

GASTROINTESTINAL MANIFESTATIONS OF SLE

Gastrointestinal manifestations have been reported in up to 40% to 60% of SLE patients. These processes have been attributed to a variety of factors including lupus-induced gastrointestinal disorders, opportunistic infections, and medication side effects (7). Severity ranges from mild symptoms to life-threatening disease, but the most common symptoms are nausea and vomiting, anorexia, and abdominal pain (8).

SLE can affect any part of the digestive system including the pancreas, gallbladder, and liver (9). SLE can also coexist with other autoimmune gastrointestinal conditions at a higher rate than seen in the normal population (9). This chapter will review a wide array of gastrointestinal syndromes that may occur in the setting of SLE including co-occurrence with other autoimmune gastrointestinal disorders, intestinal pseudo-obstruction, esophageal motility, lupus peritonitis, lupus enteritis, protein-losing enteropathy, pancreatitis associated with SLE, lupus-associated acalculous cholecystitis, and lupus hepatitis.

OCCURRENCE WITH OTHER AUTOIMMUNE GASTROINTESTINAL DISORDERS

Patients with autoimmune disorders such as lupus are at higher risk of developing additional autoimmune conditions. Primary biliary cholangitis (PBC) is an autoimmune gastrointestinal disorder that can rarely occur in SLE patients. PBC is due to an autoimmune response against intrahepatic cholangiocytes. This autoimmunity is associated with elevated levels of antimitochondrial antibodies against the mitochondrially located E2 component of the pyruvate dehydrogenase complex (10).

PBC causes cholestatic liver injury, often presenting with jaundice, pruritis from bile acids, and general fatigue (10). The estimated incidence of PBC in patients with SLE is low, ranging from 0% to 2.7%, with no clear association with the degree of SLE activity (10). Patients with both SLE and PBC appear to be almost entirely female, representing 97.1% of cases (10). PBC is most commonly associated with Sjogren's disease, not SLE, when accounting for all rheumatological diseases (11).

Celiac disease is a common autoimmune disease, with a prevalence of 1% globally (12). Celiac disease is strongly associated with type 1 diabetes mellitus and Addison's disease (12). Sjogren's is also the most common rheumatologic disorder associated with celiac disease, with a prevalence of up to 14% (12). In SLE patients, the prevalence is approximately 3%, which is higher than the prevalence in the overall population (12).

Inflammatory bowel disease (IBD) including Crohn's disease and ulcerative colitis are chronic inflammatory diseases associated with intestinal mucosal inflammation. IBD can sometimes cause extraintestinal manifestations as well. A large systematic review found that Crohn's disease but not ulcerative colitis is associated with SLE (13).

INTESTINAL PSEUDO-OBSTRUCTION

Intestinal pseudo-obstruction is due to impaired intestinal motility and, in some cases, can also involve the gastric region. Pathologically, it is thought to occur in SLE from an intestinal vasculitis leading to visceral smooth muscle and enteric nerve damage and, essentially, an autonomic nervous system dysfunction (8). Antibodies may also develop against the smooth muscle layers of the intestinal tract, directly leading to antibody-mediated damage (14). Histologically, the intestine is often edematous and inflamed with dense eosinophilic infiltration (15). Marked myocyte necrosis, myocyte loss, and atrophy or fibrosis of the muscularis propria can also be seen (15). Manometry can be helpful to clarify the diagnosis. The gastric antrum and duodenum are particularly susceptible to pseudo-obstruction (8). Pseudo-obstruction presents nearly identically to overt obstruction with nausea, abdominal distension, and abdominal pain but without any clear cause of obstruction on imaging (15). Imaging will look similar to ileus or Ogilvie syndrome with dilated small and/or large bowel loops, a thickened intestinal wall, and multiple air-fluid levels (15).

Like other gastrointestinal manifestations, intestinal pseudo-obstruction can be present both during the initial presentation of SLE and after longer-standing disease. In the United States, the estimated prevalence of intestinal pseudo-obstruction is 1.7% in SLE patients (14). In an analysis of 42 cases of pseudo-obstruction, there was a female-to-male ratio of 19:2. In this cohort, 52.4% had pseudo-obstruction present at SLE diagnosis, with the small bowel most frequently implicated (15). Most patients respond well to treatment with steroids or other immunosuppression including methotrexate, IVIG, cyclosporine, cyclophosphamide, and tacrolimus (15). Prokinetic agents such as neostigmine may be used to help increase motility, and alternative nutritional feeding such as total parenteral nutrition may be needed in cases of prolonged pseudo-obstruction (14). Surgical intervention is reserved for the most extreme scenarios (14). There is a strong risk of concomitant hydronephrosis in instances of SLE intestinal pseudo-obstruction, with up to 73.8% of SLE intestinal pseudo-obstruction of these cases described in the literature (15). This trend suggests a possible global smooth muscle injury outside of the intestines might lead to dysmotility in other organ systems such as the ureters (14, 15).

Functional intestinal obstruction, including ileus and Ogilvie syndrome, are other non–immune-mediated disorders that can present similarly to SLE-mediated intestinal pseudo-obstruction. These alternate diagnoses should be included in the diagnostic reasoning process, especially in patients who have undergone recent surgery or are on bowel-slowing medications. Ileus generally refers to impaired intestinal mobility of the small intestine leading to bowel obstruction symptoms. It is a combined mechanical and functional process, with no anatomic reason for the obstruction. Ileus is a known risk after surgery, with anesthesia side effects, sympathetic nervous system activation, and intestinal manipulation-mediated intestinal inflammation all being mechanisms of postsurgical ileus (16). Opiates, often used in the postsurgical period, are another major precipitating factor (17). Ogilvie syndrome refers to acute colonic pseudo-obstruction of sections or the entirety of the colon and rectum, often with substantial dilation (18). It most commonly occurs in patients with significantly impaired mobility and is thought to occur due to paralysis of the intestinal musculature leading to passive distension (18, 19). Pharmacological bowel slowing is also thought to play a major role, with opiates, anticholinergic medications, and calcium channel blockers being associated with Ogilvie syndrome (18). Treatment of both these entities is generally supportive including bowel rest, discontinuation of offending medications, and, in the case of refractory Ogilvie syndrome, decompression of the colon with a rectal tube (18).

ESOPHAGEAL DYSMOTILITY

Impaired esophageal peristalsis is a frequent occurrence in patients with lupus. In the United States, 1% of all patients undergoing manometry for formal evaluation of esophageal motility had background SLE (20). Esophageal dysmotility may present with chest pain, reflux, and dysphagia. In a study that performed esophageal manometry on asymptomatic SLE patients, 4 out of 25 patients had mild to moderate decreases in peristalsis with some esophageal dilation, while 1 in 25 patients were found to have aperistalsis (21). Another study of asymptomatic SLE patients found manometric abnormalities in 16 out of 50 patients (22). A third study found 50% of asymptomatic SLE patients had abnormal esophageal motility studies, though the findings were less significant than those found in mixed connective tissue disease (23). The pathophysiology is not clear but may involve an inflammatory reaction in the esophageal muscles or ischemic damage of the Auerbach plexus (24). There is also the possibility of this finding mainly occurring in patients with mixed connective tissue disorder who are misclassified as SLE or in patients who have overlap systemic sclerosis.

Treatment for esophageal dysmotility remains challenging. There are no cases of immunosuppression including prednisone being effective in the literature. Standard reflux treatment, including proton pump inhibitors or histamine H2 receptor blockers, may help reflux symptoms. However, there are no reports of this improving SLE-associated esophageal dysmotility. Metoclopramide has been used in systemic sclerosis–mediated esophageal dysmotility but has not been shown to help non–immune-mediated reflux (25, 26). It has not been formally evaluated for its efficacy in SLE.

LUPUS PERITONITIS

Lupus peritonitis is considered a subtype of serositis and involves immune-mediated inflammation of the peritoneal membrane. Lupus peritonitis may be underdiagnosed due to subclinical symptoms. Autopsy studies have shown 60% to 70% of SLE patients have findings of peritonitis, with only

10% of these cases being recognized clinically. It is worth noting the primary source of this statistic comes from a 1993 textbook that is no longer in circulation (8). Lupus peritonitis can present as pseudo-pseudo-Meigs' syndrome (27). Meigs' syndrome is the combination of ascites, pleural effusion, and elevated CA-125 seen in the setting of malignant ovarian tumors, with pseudo-Meigs' referring to this triad with a benign tumor and pseudo-pseudo-Meigs' referring to other causes such as SLE. Lupus peritonitis frequently presents with ascites clinically. However, ascites can also be a feature of other complications of SLE, including nephrotic range proteinuria, protein-losing enteropathy, and hepatitis (27). A diagnostic feature of lupus peritonitis is a low serum albumin ascites gradient compared with these other causes of ascites (27). Infection and malignancy must also be ruled out, as these can also cause ascites with a low serum albumin ascites gradient. As of 2021, 15 cases of lupus peritonitis complicated by pseudo-pseudo-Meigs' were reported, with it being the initial presentation of SLE in 50% of cases (27). A variety of agents including mycophenolate mofetil, azathioprine, rituximab, hydroxychloroquine, oral steroids, and intraperitoneal steroids were used, with a fairly robust response in most cases (27). In SLE related pseudo-pseudo-Meigs', elevated serum CA-125 levels appear to be from cytokine effects on mesothelial cells and are associated with polyserositis (27). Additionally, IL-6 levels are elevated in the ascites fluid of lupus peritonitis patients (27).

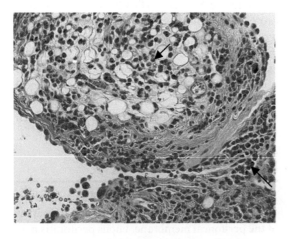

Figure 6.1 Peritoneal biopsy showing fibroadipose tissue with reactive mesothelial hyperplasia and lymphoplasmacytic infiltrate (11).

There has also been evidence of lymphoplasmacytic invasion with reactive mesothelial cell hyperplasia on peritoneal biopsies of patients (28). An example of this is shown in Figure 6.1.

LUPUS ENTERITIS

Lupus enteritis may be caused by either vasculitis or inflammation of the small bowel mucosa with supportive imaging or biopsy findings (8). Lupus mesenteric vasculitis refers to the same overarching syndrome when there are definitive histologic findings of vasculitis on biopsy (29). "Lupus enteritis" is the preferred term, as it is more inclusive, since these pathological features are only seen in a minority of cases. For example, when biopsies are performed, vasculitis is seen in 26% of cases (29). Lupus enteritis effects around 0.2% to 5.8% of SLE patients depending on the population analyzed (8). The most feared complications include bowel wall infarction, ischemia, or perforation (8). Lupus enteritis most frequently involves the jejunum and ileum (8). Macroscopic examination reveals edematous, hyperemic, or ischemic bowel with or without infarction. Histology can be nonspecific or show infiltration of the submucosal and muscular layers. Histology can also show necrotizing vasculitis that can be panmural, with predominant eosinophilic, neutrophilic, or mixed infiltrates (8, 29). The median age of onset is 34 years old, occurring 85% of the time in females, with SLE enteritis presenting on average 34.3 months after diagnosis (8).

SLE mesenteric enteritis can also be suspected based on characteristic CT imaging findings. One review of the literature found 98% of cases show bowel edema, 71% show bowel wall enhancement or the target sign, and another 71% show engorgement with increased visibility of mesenteric vessels, known as the comb sign (8, 30). These imaging findings are not pathognomonic for lupus, however, and only indicate an inflammatory process more broadly (30). Examples of the target and comb sign, respectively, can be seen in Figures 6.2 and 6.3.

The presentation of lupus enteritis may be nonspecific, comprising acute abdominal pain, fever, diarrhea, and vomiting (29). Patients tend to respond well to immunosuppression with steroids and other agents. Steroid-sparing agents have included cyclophosphamide in the acute setting, or long-term hydroxychloroquine, azathioprine,

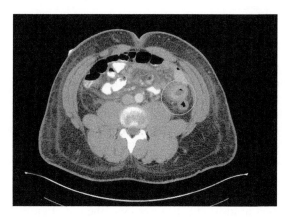

Figure 6.2 Target sign in lupus enteritis outlined in green (30).

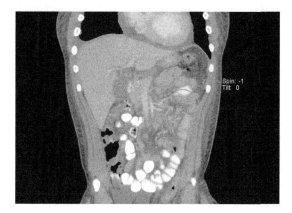

Figure 6.3 Comb sign in lupus enteritis outlined in blue (30).

and mycophenolate to prevent recurrence (29). Surgery is still sometimes required, however, with one study suggesting 11% of patients required exploratory laparotomy and 7% required bowel resection (29). It is worth noting that SLE patients may not present with classic acute features suggestive of a perforation. Thus, a high index of suspicion is needed to suspect the surgical emergency of an intestinal perforation in SLE patients (31). This subacute presentation is a result of baseline steroids or other immunosuppressants, which can decrease the inflammatory response postperforation, leading to muted symptoms (29, 31). Lupus enteritis may be a precursor to protein-losing enteropathy, with damage of the intestinal tract leading to protein leakage in some cases. However, this theory has not been analyzed in the literature. Infectious enteritis can present similarly to lupus enteritis as well and should be excluded in SLE patients presenting with these nonspecific symptoms and imaging findings.

PROTEIN-LOSING ENTEROPATHY

Protein-losing enteropathy (PLE) is a condition that results in excessive loss of serum proteins into the GI tract. This subsequently leads to hypoproteinemia, edema, pleural and pericardial effusions, diarrhea, frequent infections, and sometimes hypercoagulability due to loss of antithrombin III (32). This protein leakage occurs through one of three main mechanisms: intestinal inflammatory exudation from mucosal injury, increased intestinal mucosal permeability, and/or loss of intestinal lymphatic fluid (32). Clinically, PLE is diagnosed as the source of hypoalbuminemia based on an elevated fecal clearance of alpha-1 antitrypsin, indicating gastrointestinal leakage as the source of protein loss.

SLE-induced PLE has been reported in the literature and may be due to three proposed pathophysiologic mechanisms: vasculitis leading to increased intestinal vessel permeability, complement activation leading to cytokine-mediated damage and vasodilation, and intestinal lymphangiectasia (8). PLE often presents at the time of SLE diagnosis in association with other clinical and serological features (33). A review of cases shows the average age of presentation is 36 years old, with 66% of cases presenting at initial SLE diagnosis, 64% having mucocutaneous SLE symptoms, 14% having alopecia, 35% having lupus nephritis, 8% having Raynaud's, and 12% having neuropsychiatric involvement (34). In another review of cases, patients uniformly had low complement levels (33). Patients were also found to have other serologies including positive anti-dsDNA in 44%, anti-Sm in 11%, anti-RNP in 30%, anti-SSA in 64%, and anti-SSB in 23% of cases (34). Intestinal biopsies can be nonspecific, showing mucosal edema, inflammatory cell infiltrate, lymphangiectasia, vasculitis, and in fact, in some cases, were completely normal (33, 35). Colonoscopy may occasionally show mucosal thickening (35). Treatment of SLE-induced PLE includes immunosuppression to target the underlying SLE. Treatment is variable and has included steroids, cyclophosphamide, mycophenolate, methotrexate, IVIG, hydroxychloroquine, and azathioprine, often with good prognosis and improvement of PLE (34).

AUTOIMMUNE PANCREATITIS

Pancreatitis associated with SLE has been described in approximately 0.7% to 4% of SLE patients (8). Possible causes include vasculitis leading to tissue necrosis, antiphospholipid-associated thrombosis of pancreatic arterioles/arteries, and intimal thickening from immune complex deposition within the wall of pancreatic arteries (8). There may also be an association with SSB antibodies (8). Lupus-induced pancreatitis is poorly defined and is diagnosed only when more common etiologies are excluded including alcohol, cholelithiasis, and medications. Specifically, many medications used for SLE, especially steroids and azathioprine, can induce pancreatitis, making it difficult to differentiate drug-induced versus SLE-induced pancreatitis (36). A retrospective study of SLE-associated pancreatitis included 65.2% of patients on steroids, 9.1% on azathioprine, 7.6% on mycophenolate, and 7.6% on cyclophosphamide at baseline, demonstrating how frequently SLE patients are on concomitant medications known to induce pancreatitis (37). Steroids themselves can lead to increased viscosity of pancreatic secretions and decreased amylase and bicarbonate secretions, all contributing to the development of pancreatitis (37).

Distinguishing SLE pancreatitis from idiopathic pancreatitis or drug-induced pancreatitis remains controversial, as there are no specific diagnostic features separating these conditions. In a review of SLE patients with pancreatitis, 264 patients were analyzed using 11 articles (36). There was a high female-to-male ratio of 9:1, with an average age of 31.4 years at presentation. [Dima] Pancreatitis tended to occur 2 to 3 years after diagnosis of SLE (36). Complement levels were low in the vast majority of cases, with variable antiphospholipid positivity of 40% to 50% (36). Histologically, SLE-induced pancreatitis samples show inflammatory infiltrates and necrosis, which are indistinguishable from pancreatitis due to other causes (37).

Treatment of SLE-induced pancreatitis is variable, as is mortality, ranging anywhere from 3% to 50% in reported studies (36). In some cases, immunosuppression is associated with an improved prognosis compared to standard pancreatitis management (36). High-dose steroids, including pulse-dose steroids, IVIG, and cyclophosphamide, have been used (34, 36, 38, 39). There is also some evidence that plasma exchange may be beneficial (36, 40).

Immunosuppression is associated with a better prognosis compared to standard pancreatitis management in some cases, though in others, it has shown harm (36). For instance, a retrospective review of 46 cases showed that 4 of 8 patients treated with pulse-dose steroids and cyclophosphamide died of infections (39). In patients treated with pulse-dose steroids alone, 8 of 15 died, and of the patients treated with a combination of moderate-dose steroids and other agents, 3 of 23 died of unspecified causes (39). The use of pulse-dose steroids was significantly associated with mortality in this cohort, as was the development of infection after acute pancreatitis (39). In contrast to this, a retrospective review of 77 patients found mortality was increased in patients not treated with immunosuppression (41, 42). However, this study did not evaluate pulse-dose steroids specifically (41, 42). This discordance may be due to the difficulty in assessing whether pancreatitis is truly from SLE versus other etiologies. It may also indicate that nuances exist and that higher-intensity immunosuppression may be harmful, while more moderated intensity may be beneficial. We would favor a conservative approach to immunosuppression, particularly if there is no other evidence of a flare of lupus activity at the time of presentation.

ACALCULOUS CHOLECYSTITIS

Lupus can affect the gallbladder, leading to acalculous cholecystitis. One potential mechanism is a subclinical vasculitis damaging the biliary capillary networks (8). Other potential causes include thrombosis of gallbladder vessels in the setting of antiphospholipid antibodies that are frequently seen in SLE (43). Mesenteric inflammatory veno-occulusive disease, a vasculitis subtype involving the mesenteric veins without artery involvement, may also play a role (43). SLE-associated acalculous cholecystitis differs clinically from classic acalculous cholecystitis. Acalculous cholecystitis generally occurs in critically ill patients in the setting of hypotension, with a combination of ischemia and prolonged bile stasis causing elevated gallbladder pressures and resultant decreased blood flow (44). Conversely, SLE-associated acalculous cholecystitis is not due to critical illness. Lupus-associated acalculous cholecystitis has been reported at initial SLE presentation in approximately 30% of cases, though it generally occurs in patients with longstanding SLE (43, 45). Lupus associated acalculous cholecystitis generally responds well to treatment with steroids and hydroxychloroquine (43, 45). In a small trial, steroids plus antibiotic therapy was more effective than antibiotics alone in preventing the need for cholecystectomy, confirming the role of steroids in this condition (46). Cholecystectomy is still ultimately needed in some cases, however (43, 45).

LUPUS HEPATITIS

Liver disease is common in SLE patients and can present in a variety of ways (47). Over the course of their disease, 30% to 50% of patients develop hepatomegaly, and 25% to 50% of patients have elevated liver enzymes (47, 48). These manifestations are not all due to SLE directly and are often indirect complications from immunosuppressive therapies, especially with steroid-induced fatty liver disease (47). Liver biopsies in SLE patients showed fatty liver in 72.6%, with signs of primary biliary cholangitis (PBC) in 2.7% and autoimmune hepatitis in 2.7% of cases (47).

Autoimmune hepatitis is a separate entity from lupus hepatitis. However, there is some overlap in presentation and serologies, making it difficult to distinguish between the two conditions without biopsy. Additionally, patients with autoimmune hepatitis have a high rate of concomitant autoimmune disease. Clinically, lupus hepatitis tends to have a much better prognosis than autoimmune hepatitis, with improved survival and less progression to cirrhosis (47).

Autoimmune hepatitis can be classified by serology as type 1, type 2, or antibody negative. Type 1 antibodies can include a positive antinuclear antibody (ANA), anti–smooth muscle, antiactin, antimitochondrial, anti–soluble liver antigen/liver pancreas, atypical P-ANCA, and antisingle or antidouble stranded antibodies (49–52). Type I also includes antimitochondrial antibodies, which are associated with PBC overlap. Type 2 antibodies include antiliver kidney microsome type 1, antiliver cytosol antibody 1, and anti–soluble liver antigen/liver pancreas antibody (49–52). It is important to note that historically, type 1 autoimmune hepatitis was referred to as "lupoid hepatitis" given its ANA positivity, but this is a misnomer, as these are now classified as two separate conditions (47).

The presence of specific antibodies for autoimmune hepatitis, such as anti–smooth muscle and anti–liver-kidney microsome type 1, argues against lupus hepatitis even in a patient with concomitant lupus (47). Serological features more suggestive of lupus hepatitis include low complements and elevated anti-Sm antibodies (essentially evidence of active SLE) (47). Antiribosomal P antibodies are also associated with lupus hepatitis and are positive in 44% of cases (53).

On biopsy, lupus hepatitis generally shows lobular infiltrates or periportal infiltrates with few lymphoid cells. Autoimmune hepatitis is characterized by more aggressive inflammation with portal mononuclear infiltrates, periportal piecemeal necrosis, and rosettes of hepatocytes that can progress to lobular necrosis (47). Lupus hepatitis may also be discernable from other causes based on deposits of complement 1q on biopsy (9). Lupus hepatitis tends to respond well to steroids and treatment of the systemic disease (47). Autoimmune hepatitis is treated similarly, with azathioprine the preferred steroid-sparing agent, but some patients progress to fulminant hepatic failure regardless (54).

CONCLUSION

SLE can be associated with a wide variety of gastrointestinal symptoms and disease processes, as outlined in this chapter. These manifestations can range from toxicities associated with medications used to treat their SLE such as drug-induced pancreatitis or be a direct consequence of SLE-mediated damage to gastrointestinal organs such as lupus-associated peritonitis or acalculous cystitis. The astute clinician must be able to differentiate between lupus and other closely related diagnoses given that this will affect the treatment regimen and overall prognosis. In the future, improved understanding and identification of lupus-specific variables are needed to aid in the timely diagnosis and treatment of the gastrointestinal manifestations of SLE.

REFERENCES

1. Barber MRW, Drenkard C, Falasinnu T et al. Global epidemiology of systemic lupus erythematosus. *Nat Rev Rheumatol.* 2021;17(9):515–32.

2. Aringer M, Costenbader K, Daikh D et al. 2019 European league against rheumatism/American college of rheumatology classification criteria for systemic lupus erythematosus. *Arthritis Rheumatol.* 2019;71(9):1400–12.

3. Fanouriakis A, Kostopoulou M, Alunno A et al. 2019 update of the EULAR recommendations for the management of systemic lupus erythematosus. *Ann Rheum Dis.* 2019;78(6):736–45.

4. Plüß M, Piantoni S, Tampe B et al. Belimumab for systemic lupus erythematosus—Focus on lupus nephritis. *Hum Vaccines Immunother.* 2022;18(5).

5. Abdel-Kahaar E, Keller F. Clinical pharmacokinetics and pharmacodynamics of dalbavancin. *Clin Pharmacokinet.* 2023;62(5):693–703.

6. Niebel D, de Vos L, Fetter T et al. Cutaneous lupus erythematosus: An update on pathogenesis and future therapeutic directions. *Am J Clin Dermatol.* 2023;(0123456789).

7. Frittoli RB, Vivaldo JF, Costallat LTL et al. Gastrointestinal involvement in systemic lupus erythematosus: A systematic review. *J Transl Autoimmun.* 2021 Jun;4:1–9.

8. Brewer B, Kamen D. Gastrointestinal and hepatic disease in systemic lupus erythematosus. *Rheum Dis Clin North Am.* 2018;44(1):165–75.

9. Alharbi S. Gastrointestinal manifestations in patients with systemic lupus erythematosus. *Open Access Rheumatol Res Rev.* 2022 Oct;14:243–53.

10. Shizuma T. Clinical characteristics of concomitant systemic lupus erythematosus and primary biliary cirrhosis: A literature review. *J Immunol Res.* 2015;2015.

11. Efe C, Torgutalp M, Henriksson I et al. Extrahepatic autoimmune diseases in primary biliary cholangitis: Prevalence and significance for clinical presentation and disease outcome. *J Gastroenterol Hepatol.* 2021;36(4):936–42.

12. Soltani Z, Baghdadi A, Nejadhosseinian M et al. Celiac disease in patients with systemic lupus erythematosus. *Reumatologia.* 2021;59(2):85–9.

13. Shor DBA, Dahan S, Comaneshter D et al. Does inflammatory bowel disease coexist with systemic lupus erythematosus? *Autoimmun Rev.* 2016;15(11):1034–7.

14. Zheng J, Ni R, Liu H. Intestinal pseudo-obstruction in systemic lupus erythematosus: An analysis of nationwide inpatient sample. *Clin Rheumatol.* 2022;41(11):3331–5.

15. Jin P, Ji X, Zhi H et al. A review of 42 cases of intestinal pseudo-obstruction in patients with systemic lupus erythematosus based on case reports. *Hum Immunol.* 2015;76(9):695–700.

16. Venara A, Neunlist M, Slim K et al. Postoperative ileus: Pathophysiology, incidence, and prevention. *J Visc Surg.* 2016;153(6):439–46.

17. Buscail E, Deraison C. Postoperative ileus: A pharmacological perspective. *Br J Pharmacol.* 2022;179(13):3283–305.

18. Pereira P, Djeudji F, Leduc P et al. Ogilvie's syndrome—Acute colonic pseudo-obstruction. *J Chir Viscerale.* 2015;152(2):99–105.

19. Haj M, Haj M, Rockey DC. Ogilvie's syndrome : Management and outcomes. *Med (Baltimore).* 2018;97(17):1–6.

20. Turshudzhyan A, Abbasi AF, Banerjee P. Hidden in plain sight: Esophageal dysmotility in patients with systemic lupus erythematosus. *Cureus.* 2022;14(Ild):3–5.

21. Tatelman M, Keech M. Esophageal motility in systemic lupus erythematosus, rheumatoid arthritis, and scleroderma. *Radiol Soc North Am.* 1966;86(6):1041–6.

22. Ramirez-Mata M, Reyes PA, Alarcon-Segovia D et al. Esophageal motility in systemic lupus erythematosus. *Am J Dig Dis.* 1974;19(2):132–6.

23. Gutierrez F, Valenzuela J, Ehresmann G et al. Esophageal dysfunction in patients with progressive systemic sclerosis and mixed connective tissue diseases. *Dig Dis Sci.* 1982;27(7):592–7.

24. Castrucci G, Alimandi L, Fichera A et al. Changes in esophageal motility in patients with systemic lupus erythematosus: An esophago-manometric study. *Minerva Dietol Gastroenterol.* 1990;36(1):3–7.

25. Sridhar KR, Lange RC, Magyar L et al. Prevalence of impaired gastric emptying of

solids in systemic sclerosis: Diagnostic and therapeutic implications. *J Lab Clin Med.* 1998;132(6):541–6.

26. Grande L, Lacima G, Ros E et al. Lack of effect of metoclopramide and domperidone on esophageal peristalsis and esophageal acid clearance in reflux esophagitis—A randomized, double-blind study. *Dig Dis Sci.* 1992;37(4):583–8.

27. Meena DS, Kumar B, Gopalakrishnan M et al. Pseudo—Pseudo Meigs' Syndrome (PPMS) in chronic lupus peritonitis: A case report with review of literature. *Mod Rheumatol Case Rep.* 2021;5(2):300–5.

28. Dalvi SR, Yildirim R, Santoriello D et al. Pseudo-pseudo Meigs' syndrome in a patient with systemic lupus erythematosus. *Lupus.* 2012;21(13):1463–6.

29. Janssens P, Arnaud L, Galicier L et al. Lupus enteritis: From clinical findings to therapeutic management. *Orphanet J Rare Dis.* 2013;8(1):1–10.

30. Faraji M, Gutierrez E, Glotser A et al. Targets and combs: A case of lupus enteritis. *Cureus.* 2020;12(4):10–13.

31. Spencer SP, Power N. The acute abdomen in the immune compromised host. *Cancer Imaging.* 2008;8(1):93–101.

32. Levitt DG, Levitt MD. Protein losing enteropathy: Comprehensive review of the mechanistic association with clinical and subclinical disease states. *Clin Exp Gastroenterol.* 2017;10:147–68.

33. Perednia DA, Curosh NA. Lupus-associated protein-losing enteropathy. *Arch Intern Med.* 1990;150(1):1806–10.

34. Li Z, Xu D, Wang Z et al. Gastrointestinal system involvement in systemic lupus erythematosus. *Lupus.* 2017;26(11):1127–38.

35. Al-mogairen SM. Lupus Protein-Losing Enteropathy (LUPLE): A systematic review. *Rheumatol Int.* 2011;31:995–1001.

36. Dima A, Balaban DV, Jurcut C et al. Systemic lupus erythematosus-related acute pancreatitis. *Lupus.* 2021;30(1):5–14.

37. Muhammed H, Jain A, Irfan M et al. Clinical features, severity and outcome of acute pancreatitis in systemic lupus erythematosus. *Rheumatol Int.* 2022;42(8):1363–71.

38. Ben Dhaou B, Aydi Z, Boussema F et al. La pancréatite lupique: une série de six cas. *La Rev Médecine Interne.* 2013 Jan 1;34(1):12–16.

39. Wang Q, Shen M, Leng X et al. Prevalence, severity, and clinical features of acute and chronic pancreatitis in patients with systemic lupus erythematosus. *Rheumatol Int.* 2016;36(10):1413–19.

40. Yu Y-K, Yu F, Ye C et al. Retrospective analysis of plasma exchange combined with glucocorticosteroids for the treatment of systemic lupus erythematosus-related acute pancreatitis in central China. *J Huazhong Univ Sci Technol—Med Sci.* 2016;36(4):501–8.

41. Nesher G, Breuer GS, Temprano K et al. Lupus-associated pancreatitis. *Semin Arthritis Rheum.* 2006;35(4):260–7.

42. Breuer GS, Baer A, Dahan D et al. Lupus-associated pancreatitis. *Autoimmun Rev.* 2006;5(5):314–18.

43. Lee J, Lee YJ, Kim Y. Acute acalculous cholecystitis as the initial manifestation of systemic lupus erythematous: A case report. *Med (Baltimore).* 2021;100(22):e26238.

44. Fu Y, Pang L, Dai W et al. Advances in the study of acute acalculous cholecystitis: A comprehensive review. *Dig Dis.* 2022;40(4):468–78.

45. Yang H, Bian S, Xu D et al. Acute acalculous cholecystitis in patients with systemic lupus erythematosus: A unique form of disease flare. *Lupus.* 2017;26(10):1101–5.

46. Liu W, Chen W, He X et al. Successful treatment using corticosteroid combined antibiotic for acute acalculous cholecystitis patients with systemic lupus erythematosus. *Med* (United States). 2017;96(27).

47. Adiga A, Nugent K. Lupus hepatitis and autoimmune hepatitis (lupoid hepatitis). *Am J Med Sci* [Internet]. 2017;353(4):329–35. http://doi.org/10.1016/j.amjms.2016.10.014

48. van Hoek B. The spectrum of liver disease in systemic lupus erythematosus. *Neth J Med.* 1996;48(6):244–53.

49. Terjung B, Spengler U, Sauerbruch T et al. "Atypical p-ANCA" in IBD and hepatobiliary disorders react with a 50-kilodalton nuclear envelope protein of neutrophils

and myeloid cell lines. *Gastroenterol.* 2000;119(2):310–22.

50. Mack CL, Adams D, Assis DN et al. Diagnosis and management of autoimmune hepatitis in adults and children: 2019 practice guidance and guidelines from the American association for the study of liver diseases. *Hepatol.* 2020;72(2):671–722.

51. Czaja AJ, Carpenter HA, Manns MP. Antibodies to soluble liver antigen, P450IID6, and mitochondrial complexes in chronic hepatitis. *Gastroenterol.* 1993 Nov 1;105(5):1522–8.

52. Czaja AJ, Morshed SA, Parveen S et al. Antibodies to single-stranded and double-stranded DNA in antinuclear antibody-positive type 1-autoimmune hepatitis. *Hepatol.* 1997;26(3):567–72.

53. Ohira H, Takiguchi J, Rai T et al. High frequency of anti-ribosomal P antibody in patients with systemic lupus erythematosus-associated hepatitis. *Hepatol Res.* 2004 Mar 1;28(3):137–9.

54. Lohse AW, Chazouillères O, Dalekos G et al. EASL clinical practice guidelines: Autoimmune hepatitis. *J Hepatol.* 2015;63(4):971–1004.

7

Scleroderma and Myositis

RAWISH FATIMA AND NEZAM ALTOROK

SCLERODERMA

Scleroderma is an immune-mediated chronic multiorgan disease whose etiology remains largely unknown. It is characterized by widespread microvascular damage with excessive collagen deposition. It affects women more than men, and the typical age of presentation is between ages 30 and 50.

CLASSIFICATION

'Scleroderma' is an umbrella term that includes both localized scleroderma, which is a fibrotic disease limited to the skin with no other organ involvement, and systemic sclerosis—where the term indicates a systemic disease with additional organ involvement. Table 7.1 provides a summary of classification of scleroderma.

Table 7.1 Summary of Classification of Scleroderma

Categories of scleroderma	Types of each category
Localized scleroderma/ morphea	1. Circumscribed morphea 2. Generalized morphea 3. Linear scleroderma
Systemic scleroderma/ systemic sclerosis	1. Limited scleroderma (LcSSc) 2. Diffuse scleroderma (DcSSc) 3. Sine sclerosis (ssSSc)

There are three types of *localized scleroderma*.

1. Circumscribed morphea (Figure 7.1) are discolored patches of skin that can vary in size and typically have red borders with a thickened pale-yellow center. The lesions enlarge when they are active and flatten and become asymptomatic with treatment. Oftentimes, deep circumscribed morphea can extend into subcutaneous tissue.
2. Generalized morphea is the presence of several patches of morphea (greater than four plaques in many anatomical areas). They can blend into each other and form pansclerotic morphea, which is a severe form of generalized morphea that involves most of the body.
3. Linear scleroderma. These are tight, thick bands that can appear on extremities, trunk, buttocks, or face. When it appears on the arms or legs, it can affect the development of a child's limb, causing disability (1–3).

Systemic sclerosis (SSc) is classified into three groups based on the extent of skin involvement:

1. Limited cutaneous systemic sclerosis (lcSS), where skin fibrosis is limited to skin distal to elbows and knees. Of note, CREST syndrome (C: calcinosis, R: Raynaud's phenomenon, E: esophageal dysmotility, S: sclerodactyly, T: telangiectasia) was used to describe lcSS, but the term CREST is obsolete now, as not all patients with lcSS will have all manifestations of CREST.

DOI: 10.1201/9781003367307-7

2. Diffuse cutaneous systemic sclerosis (dcSS), which has truncal and acral skin involvement proximal to elbows and knees.
3. Systemic sclerosis sine scleroderma (ssSSc) is a third subset that is much less common, where there are features of systemic disease and organ involvement with no skin disease.

There have also been reports of scleroderma overlap syndromes, in which two or more consecutive connective tissue disorders exist in the same patient. The frequency of these syndromes in scleroderma is 10% to 38% based on available data. The common overlapping syndromes are polymyalgia rheumatica, rheumatoid arthritis (RA), systemic lupus erythematosus (SLE) -overlap (4).

Of interest, there is an entity of 'pre-scleroderma' or 'very early SSc' characterized by Raynaud's phenomenon, puffy fingers, nailfold capillary changes, evidence of digital ischemia, and presence of either specific SSc autoantibodies (anticentromere, anti-topoisomerase I, anti-RNA polymerase III, anti-fibrillarin or anti-Th/To) or positive anti-nuclear antibodies (ANA) with nucleolar immunofluorescence pattern. In 2011, criteria for very early diagnosis of SSc (VEDOSS) was proposed. It is a good tool for evaluation of patients who may progress to develop SSc, as per the 2013 ACR-EULAR criteria, within 5 years of follow-up. The presence of Raynaud's phenomenon, puffy fingers, and positive ANA are the red flags that lead to the suspicion of very early SSc. Abnormal nailfold capillaroscopy or SSc-associated antibodies lead to the diagnosis of very early systemic sclerosis and warrant further systemic workup and close monitoring (5).

PATHOGENESIS

The etiology and pathogenesis of localized scleroderma and systemic sclerosis are incompletely understood. It is thought that there is a genetic predisposition to these conditions. An exposure to environmental factor(s) triggers a cascade of inflammatory reactions and activates tissue fibrosis. It is hypothesized that the initial inflammatory injury is localized to the microvascular endothelial cells (6). No specific genetic alterations have been identified in morphea, but these patients have high rates of autoimmune disease in their families. Some of the environmental factors that have been postulated to contribute to the development of morphea include Lyme disease, trauma, radiation, medications, and viral infections.

Several studies have revealed the association of systemic sclerosis with HLA class II gene region, IRF5, CD247, BANK1, STAT4, TNFSF4, and BLK genes. In systemic sclerosis, postulated environmental factors include exposure to vinyl chloride, silica dust and organic solvents, medications (bleomycin, pentazocine, cocaine), and viruses (cytomegalovirus, parvovirus B19) (1, 2).

PRESENCE OF AUTOANTIBODIES

Antibodies in scleroderma are not known to play a role in pathogenesis of the disease but are used as markers of clinical, genetic and etiologic classification. They are associated with different clinical manifestations and genetic features and may ultimately further our understanding of this disease.

Over 95% of patients with systemic sclerosis have a positive ANA, compared to 20% to 80% of morphea cases. Other antibodies that are almost exclusively found in patients with systemic sclerosis are anticentromere antibodies, antitopoisomerase I (anti-Scl 70) antibodies, and anti-RNA

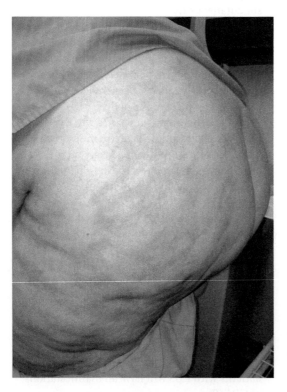

Figure 7.1 Circumscribed morphea.

polymerase III antibodies. Anti–single-stranded antibodies, antihistone antibodies, and antitopoisomerase II-α antibodies were more commonly found in patients with morphea than patients with systemic sclerosis (7, 8).

CLINICAL RELEVANCE OF AUTOANTIBODIES

Significant serologic heterogeneity is seen in SSc. The relationship between presence of autoantibodies and their role in pathogenesis remains controversial, but these serologic markers are useful in the diagnosis and clinical management of scleroderma patients. Table 7.2 summarizes the clinical significance of each SSc-specific/associated antibody.

RNA: ribonucleic acid; RNP: ribonucleoprotein; PM-Scl: polymyalgia-scleroderma; MCTD: mixed connective tissue disease; Anti-hUBF (NOR 90): antihuman upstream binding factor (autoantibodies against nucleolar organizing regions); Anti-Ro52/TRIM21: anti-Ro52/tripartite motif-containing protein 21 (9, 10).

SYSTEMIC INVOLVEMENT

Skin Involvement

Skin involvement in SSc initially starts as puffy fingers due to microvascular injury and inflammation, leading to capillary leak in the interstitial space. Collagen deposition over time leads to skin thickening and joint contractures. Of interest,

Table 7.2 Summary of autoantibodies and their clinical associations in systemic sclerosis

Autoantibodies	Disease subtype	Clinical association	Prognosis
Anti-RNA polymerase III	dcSSc	Renal crisis Increased cancer risk	Increased mortality
Anti-U11/U12 RNP		Raynaud's phenomenon	Increased mortality
Anti-Th/To	lcSSc	Pulmonary fibrosis, small bowel involvement, hypothyroidism, and renal crisis	Poor prognosis
Anti-Scl-70	dcSSc	Pulmonary fibrosis	Poor prognosis
AFA, antifibrillarin/ Anti-U3RNP	dcSSc	Renal crisis and cardiac involvement	Poor prognosis especially in African-Americans
Anticentromere	lcSSc	Pulmonary arterial hypertension	Better prognosis
Anti-U1-RNP	lcSSc	Raynaud's phenomenon, puffy fingers, arthritis, myositis, overlap syndrome (i.e., MCTD)	Better prognosis
Anti-PM-Scl	lcSSc	Raynaud's phenomenon, arthritis, myositis, pulmonary involvement, calcinosis, and sicca symptoms	Better prognosis
Anti-hUBF (NOR 90)	lcSSc	Mild internal organ involvement	Better prognosis
Anti-Ku	Overlap syndrome with scleroderma features	Myositis, arthritis, and joint contractures	
Anti-Ro52/TRIM21		Older age onset, pulmonary fibrosis	

skin involvement in dcSS tends to be worse in the early phases of the disease onset, and mRSS may improve spontaneously in the late phases of dcSSc.

Lung Involvement

All patients diagnosed with systemic sclerosis should be screened for interstitial lung disease. It is most often seen in dcSSc, especially those who are male, who are African American, or who have comorbid digital ulcerations or pulmonary hypertension on echocardiogram. Antitopoisomerase (anti-Scl 70) is an additional risk factor. The most frequent imaging pattern on high-resolution CT (HRCT) is nonspecific interstitial pneumonia (NSIP). Restrictive lung disease due to restricted chest wall movement from advanced skin disease is a rarer cause of respiratory failure. Treatment for ILD includes antifibrotic agents like nintedanib in patients with a predominantly fibrotic pattern on CT chest. The use of immunosuppressive therapy for ILD with either mycophenolate or, more rarely, cyclophosphamide are typically first-line therapies in patients with a more inflammatory disease phenotype. Combination therapy and newer agents like tocilizumab may also be options in selected sub-groups of patients depending on their disease characteristics.

Renal Involvement

The pathogenesis of scleroderma renal crisis (SRC) is not completely understood, but abnormal and excessive activation of the renin-angiotensin-aldosterone system plays an important role. Renal biopsy will show typical arterial 'onion-skin' lesions, with fibrin deposits found in the thickened intima. These patients often present with malignant hypertension, hypertensive encephalopathy, congestive heart failure, and microangiopathic hemolytic anemia. Prompt recognition of SRC is of prime importance, as these patients can be successfully treated with angiotensin-converting enzyme inhibitors, and mortality is higher with delayed diagnosis (7, 10).

Cardiac Involvement

Patients can rarely develop myocarditis, congestive heart failure, arrythmia, asymptomatic focal fibrosis, and impaired ventricular relaxation. Electrocardiogram, echocardiogram, and MRI are the tools used for evaluating these patients. Such cardiac complications remain uncommon but signal a particularly poor prognosis

Pulmonary Arterial Hypertension

Patients with systemic sclerosis–associated pulmonary arterial hypertension have higher degree of mortality than those in whom this process is spared. It is more commonly seen in people with anti-centromere antibodies, Th/To autoantibodies, extensive telangiectasias, and longer disease duration (7, 11). Early recognition and prompt initiation of vasodilator therapies are important for improving survival.

Musculoskeletal Involvement

Restricted range of motion due to joint contractures, erosive arthritis, and myopathy are some of the symptoms that these patients experience. The overlap with myositis can often lead to elevated creatinine kinase levels but with a less aggressive phenotype (7).

Prognosis

Morphea does not lead to an increase in mortality but significantly increases morbidity. Children who have morphea on the head and neck are at increased risk of having neurologic and ocular involvement and need to be seen by an ophthalmologist regularly. Adults with morphea do not seem to have associated comorbidities but have an increased risk of developing concomitant autoimmune disorders (1).

Systemic sclerosis has the highest mortality among all autoimmune connective tissue diseases. Most of the increased mortality in systemic sclerosis is due to cardiopulmonary involvement (interstitial lung disease and pulmonary artery hypertension). Median survival in systemic sclerosis after diagnosis of pulmonary artery hypertension drops to 2 years and, after diagnosis of interstitial lung disease, is less than 5 years. Therefore, annual screening and early intervention are of utmost importance in these patients.

Patients with systemic sclerosis may develop serious complications in pregnancy like pulmonary hypertension, congestive heart failure, ventricular arrhythmias, and milder issues such as gastroesophageal reflux. There was also an increased incidence of intrauterine growth retardation, miscarriages, small-for-gestational-age newborns, preeclampsia, and premature deliveries. Therefore, these patients require pre-pregnancy counseling and close monitoring by a multidisciplinary team (12, 13). There have been case studies evaluating outcomes in patients with morphea that suggest that most of these patients do not experience exacerbation of disease during pregnancy (14).

Features	Subfeatures	Scores
Raynaud's phenomenon		
Pulmonary arterial hypertension	Pulmonary arterial HTN	2
	LLD	2
Presence of SSc related antibodies	Anticentromere	2
	Antitopoisomerase 1	
	Anti RNA polymerase III	

Diagnosis

The clinical presentation of SSc can be variable due to the diversity of organ and tissue involvement. In general, the majority of patients with SSc will present with (i) Raynaud's phenomenon that predates the onset of skin fibrosis, (ii) sclerodactyly, and (iii) positive ANA or SSc-specific antibodies. It is recommended that all patients with SSc should undergo pulmonary function test, CT scan of the lungs, and echocardiography to evaluate for ILD and pulmonary hypertension. Other tests that are necessary to evaluate the extent of SSc should be considered based on symptoms of organ involvement such as electrocardiogram (EKG or ECG), upper endoscopy, and gastrointestinal motility studies.

Classification Criteria

In 2013, the American College of Rheumatology/European League Against Rheumatism (ACR/EULAR) introduced a new criterion. The total score is determined by adding the maximum score the patient gets in each category, and a total score of 9 is classified as having SSc (15).

Features	Subfeatures	Scores
Skin thickening proximal to MCP		9
Skin thickening of fingers	Puffy fingers	2
	Sclerodactyly	4
Fingertip lesions	Digital tip ulcers	2
	Fingertip pitting scar	3
Telangiectasia		2
Abnormal nailfold capillary		

Treatment

In systemic sclerosis, the treatment depends on the disease comorbidities. Patients experiencing Raynaud's phenomenon should be started on dihydropyridine calcium channel blockers. When these patients develop digital ulcerations, adding sildenafil, bosentan, or even intravenous iloprost can be helpful.

Patients experiencing symptoms of myositis, arthritis, or overlap syndromes are treated with methotrexate or azathioprine. Generally, skin involvement can be at least partially responsive to treatment with mycophenolate mofetil or methotrexate. For ILD, cyclophosphamide or mycophenolate is recommended. Tocilizumab, and IL-6 antagonist, can be useful as an add-on therapy for SSc-ILD (16).

Similar to systemic sclerosis, treatment of morphea depends on the subtype, areas involved, and disease activity. Active morphea is treated with topical or systemic immunosuppressive agents, but they are of no use in burnt-out disease. Limited superficial plaque morphea is best treated with topical therapy with tacrolimus, imiquimod, combination of calcipotriol and betamethasone, or local phototherapy. Deep plaque morphea may also require phototherapy. If systemic immunosuppression is required, a combination of methotrexate and steroid taper is recommended. Phototherapy that has been reported to show improvement includes narrowband ultraviolet (UV) B, UVA, low- and medium-dose UVA1, and psoralen plus UVA (PUVA).

Linear morphea in children needs aggressive treatment with methotrexate and steroid taper. Given the in vitro and in vivo antifibrotic properties of mycophenolate mofetil, it is used as a second-line agent for patients who fail or have contraindications to methotrexate (2, 7).

Gastrointestinal Involvement in Systemic Sclerosis

Gastrointestinal (GI) tract involvement of SSc is the most common cause of morbidity in SSc and the third-most-common cause of mortality: almost every patient will have some level of symptomatic GI disease. Dysmotility is the hallmark of SSc in the GI tract. The clinical presentation of GI disease appears to vary based on SSc subtypes. For instance, fecal incontinence and meteorism (gas accumulation in GI tract leading to discomfort) were more frequently reported by patients with lcSSc, whereas nighttime heartburn, daytime heartburn, stomachache, and diarrhea were commonly reported by patients with dcSSc (17).

Mechanism of SSc-GI Disease

There is a complex interplay of vascular dysregulation, immunologic alterations, inflammation, and increased fibrinogenesis in the pathogenesis of gastrointestinal manifestations of systemic sclerosis.

It is suggested that some genetic components play a part in the initial events. Physical and chemical stimuli are then postulated to propagate this damage and may include gadolinium, L-tryptophan, cigarette smoking, organisms such as *Helicobacter pylori*, some viruses, and fungal infections.

A loss of balance between vasodilator and vasoconstrictor mechanisms is seen in these patients, which causes inappropriate vasoconstriction. At the same time, a procoagulant state is generated by the presence of adhesion molecules, which, along with increased platelet aggregation and fibrin deposition, causes formation of intravascular thrombi. As the disease advances, vascular architecture is further lost, with further resultant hypoxic and ischemic changes.

Once there is diffuse microvascular endothelial injury, an alteration of the immune microenvironment takes place. Recruitment of macrophages, lymphocytes, and cytokines like TGF-beta production causes transformation of fibroblasts to myofibroblasts, which then leads to tissue fibrosis within the GI tract (18, 19).

CLINICAL MANIFESTATIONS AND MANAGEMENT

Oral Cavity

Skin fibrosis around the oral cavity can lead to loss of skin wrinkling around the mouth, retraction of lips, and decreased oral aperture (microstomia), which leads to difficulty with pronunciation and mastication and poor dental hygiene. The incidence of tongue and oral cavity squamous cell carcinomas also is higher in SSc than in the normal population. It is recommended to obtain regular intraoral examinations to maintain oral hygiene and monitor for nonhealing oral lesions (20).

Patients with secondary Sjogren's need to seek adequate dental care and maintain salivary flow where possible. Interventions like cevimeline, pilocarpine, muscarinic agonists, and artificial saliva can be used to this end.

Esophagus

Esophageal involvement is extremely common in SSc. Symptoms include dysphagia, gastrointestinal reflux disease (GERD), odynophagia, chronic cough, hoarseness, and regurgitation due to absent or ineffective peristalsis and hypotensive lower esophageal sphincter pressure. If GERD is not adequately controlled, interstitial lung disease may be promoted as a result of lung irritation from chronic microaspiration of gastric acid (21). There is a higher risk for developing esophageal strictures and Barrett's esophagus in SSc, with the latter being a major risk factor for esophageal adenocarcinoma.

Esophagogastroduodenoscopy (EGD), manometry, and esophageal PH monitoring can be useful tests in these patients to confirm origin of these symptoms. Studies have shown that early detection and management improves outcomes.

Management of esophageal disease in SSc requires a combination of lifestyle modifications that includes weight loss, avoidance of aggravating foods, alcohol, tobacco products, and having meals a few hours before bedtime and interventions like acid suppression with proton pump inhibitors (PPIs) or H2 blockers to control their GERD. The use of antihistamines should be weighed carefully in individuals experiencing xerostomia. In resistant GERD, higher-dose proton pump inhibitors +/- combination with H2 blockers can be recommended. Using prokinetic drugs, like cisapride, domperidone, and metoclopramide, may be effective in improving gastric emptying, esophageal sphincter pressure, and intestinal peristalsis. However, use of these agents is limited by side effects. Some patients require frequent endoscopic dilation for esophageal strictures.

Stomach

Gastroparesis can be one of the more distressing complications of SSc. The clinical presentation of gastroparesis includes early satiety, recurrent nausea/vomiting, abdominal pain, bloating, and distention. Gastric emptying via scintigraphy is used for diagnosis. Lifestyle modification with the consumption of smaller meals and avoidance of foods that aggravate symptoms is always the initial therapy. Promotility agents such as metoclopramide and erythromycin also may be used. Invasive procedures, such as a jejunostomy tube or gastrostomy tube for feeding and gastric decompression, are considered in patients who experience refractory symptoms despite pharmacotherapy. Laparoscopic or endoscopic pyloroplasty rarely needs to be performed for managing gastroparesis.

Gastric antral vascular ectasia (GAVE), gastritis, and gastric ulcers can also be associated with SSc. GAVE presents as multiple longitudinal columns of red vessels, giving the characteristic "watermelon stomach" appearance on endoscopic examination. The etiology of GAVE remains poorly understood due to a paucity of studies, but it has been postulated to be a manifestation of microangiopathy of SSc (22, 23). In general, vasculopathy is considered one of the hallmarks of SSc where there is evidence of microvascular endothelial cell (MVEC) dysfunction as the most fundamental and earliest pathological lesion in SSc (25). SSc vasculopathy is associated with progressive endothelial damage, reduction in the number of capillaries, thickening of arteriolar walls, and disorganized angiogenesis, which may lead to vascular ectasia. GAVE should be suspected in patients experiencing symptomatic anemia or evidence of chronic occult gastrointestinal bleeding. Initial management by supportive measures like iron supplementation, intravenous fluids, and blood transfusion is recommended, followed by endoscopic coagulation with laser therapy, argon plasma coagulation, and endoscopic band ligation. In refractory cases, radiofrequency intervention may be needed. Figure 7.2 summarizes the upper gastrointestinal involvement that can manifest in systemic sclerosis. Figure 7.3 describes a proposed diagnostic algorithm for these symptom.

Liver

Systemic sclerosis may be associated with autoimmune liver disease, most commonly primary biliary cholangitis (PBC), followed by autoimmune hepatitis (AIH). The early signs and symptoms to seek for development of PBC include pruritis, fatigue, and elevation of alkaline phosphatase on laboratory testing. Studies have shown slower progression as compared to patients who have PBC alone. A combination of antimitochondrial antibody (AMA) and anti-sp100 can be used for screening. Often, when the antibodies are negative, liver biopsy can be performed for diagnosis. Ursodeoxycholic acid (UDCA) is the treatment of choice, and liver transplant is recommended for patients in advanced-stage disease.

AIH is suspected if patients have elevated gamma globulins (IgG), liver histology supporting inflammatory hepatitis in the absence of viral hepatitis, and presence of antibodies: antinuclear antibodies (ANA), soluble liver antigen/liver pancreas antibodies (SLA/LP), smooth muscle antibodies (SMA), or liver/kidney microsomal antibody (LKM). Treatment consists of an immunosuppressive regimen that often includes prednisolone and azathioprine.

Pancreas

Pancreatic involvement in SSc is rare and usually represents exocrine insufficiency that may not be clinically significant. Pancreatic insufficiency can mimic small intestinal bacterial overgrowth (SIBO) symptomatically, as the presentation can include diarrhea and bloating. Pancreatic

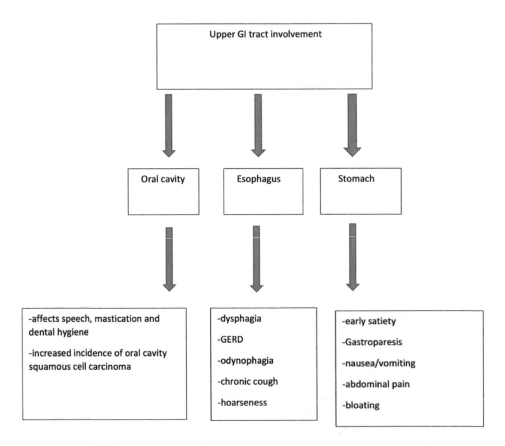

Figure 7.2 Summary of upper gastrointestinal complications of scleroderma.

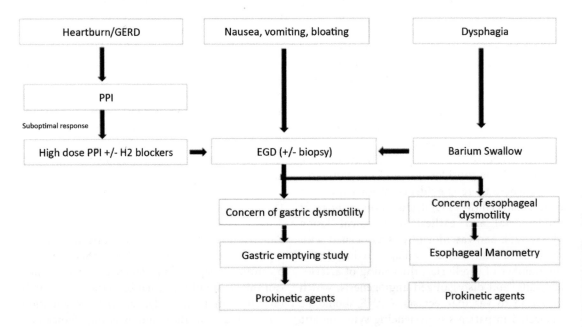

Figure 7.3 A proposed diagnostic approach for upper gastrointestinal symptoms in systemic sclerosis. Reproduced with permission (24).

insufficiency should be suspected in patients who do not respond to treatment with empiric antibiotics and have abnormal fecal fat testing. Pancreatic enzyme replacement is suggested in these cases.

Small Intestine

Small intestine involvement often presents as small intestinal bacterial overgrowth (SIBO), pseudo-obstruction, nutritional deficiency, malnutrition, and weight loss.

SIBO: Hydrogen (glucose or lactulose) and methane breath tests are used to diagnose SIBO. It has 60% sensitivity and 80% specificity, making it a favorable diagnostic option for SIBO assessment. Patients with SIBO are often empirically treated with cyclic antibiotics (like rifaximin, ciprofloxacin, norfloxacin, metronidazole, or trimethoprim-sulfamethoxazole) for a duration of 10 to 14 days based on the severity of reported symptoms (26, 27). The role of probiotics in managing bacterial overgrowth syndrome is a rapidly evolving field, and studies are underway to assess their clinical effectiveness.

Intestinal pseudo-obstruction: Patients experiencing pseudo-obstruction are often hospitalized with the aim to provide bowel rest, decompression with a nasogastric tube, intravenous fluids, broad-spectrum antibiotics, and correction of electrolyte imbalances. Cross-sectional imaging of the small intestine is the method of choice to evaluate pseudo-obstruction in the abdomen and is managed by administering prokinetic agents if conservative management fails.

Colon

Colonic dysmotility most often presents with symptoms of constipation and recurrent pseudo-obstruction. Stimulant laxatives and stool softeners along with prokinetic agents, including prucalopride, are used for management of constipation in SSc.

Chronic intestinal pseudo-obstruction (CIPO) is diagnosed through radiographic and manometric modalities. Surgical intervention is considered the last resort if conservative managements fail to improve symptoms. In severe cases, total parenteral nutrition may be needed to bypass the GI tract entirely.

The differential diagnoses for diarrhea in SSc include bile acid malabsorption, *Clostridium difficile* infection, fructose intolerance, SIBO, and amyloidosis. The treatment is guided by etiology. The first-line therapy includes dietary modification or targeted dietary therapy based on FODMAP administration (fermentable oligosaccharides, disaccharides, monosaccharides, and polyols). Use of loperamide in selective cases can also assists in managing diarrhea in patients with SSc (27).

Anorectum

It is hypothesized that anorectal dysfunction in SSc is caused by thinning, atrophy, and fibrosis of the internal anal sphincter and absence of recto-anal inhibitory reflex. This is accompanied by higher anal sensory threshold which can contribute to the development of fecal incontinence in SSc (28). Fecal incontinence may affect up to 50% of patients with SSc during their disease course and is associated with significantly reduced quality of life.

Constipation and rectal prolapse can also develop later in the course of disease (29). Standard treatments for anorectal involvement in SSc include pelvic physical therapy and biofeedback. Accumulating data from small studies suggests that posterior tibial nerve stimulation (PTNS) may benefit SSc patients with fecal incontinence who fail conservative therapy (30). Figure 7.4 summarizes the lower gastrointestinal involvement that can manifest in systemic sclerosis and figure 7.5 highlights a proposed diagnostic algorithm.

CONCLUSION

GI involvement in systemic sclerosis is varied, occurring at multiple levels of the GI tract and with considerable challenges in management. A collaborative GI–rheumatology approach is needed, and the patient's social and psychological factors should not be neglected, as there is substantial impact on quality of life.

MYOSITIS

Myositis or idiopathic inflammatory myopathies is a group of conditions that presents with symmetric proximal muscle weakness. It includes dermatomyositis (DM), polymyositis (PM), necrotizing

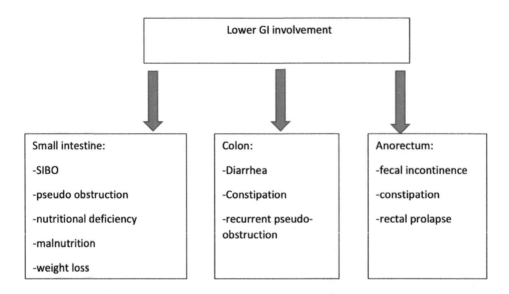

Figure 7.4 Summary of lower gastrointestinal complications of scleroderma.

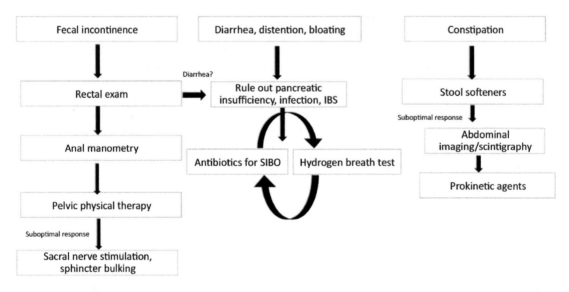

Figure 7.5 A proposed diagnostic approach for lower gastrointestinal symptoms in systemic sclerosis. Reproduced with permission (24).

myopathy (NM), and inclusion body myositis (IBM). IBM has more distal muscle involvement and a poorer response to immunosuppression than the other subtypes. An overview of each type of myositis is given in what follows

Dermatomyositis (DM)

DM tends to affect women more than men, and it has a higher prevalence in older age groups. The most common clinical presentation is symmetric proximal weakness developing within weeks to months along with an erythematous skin rash in stereotypical patterns. These skin changes can either precede or follow myopathy. Typical signs include heliotrope rash, eyelid edema, mechanic's hands, Gottron papules, less frequently myalgias, and, in severe cases, dysphagia. DM is known to have a variety of extramacular manifestations, including dysphagia, dysarthria, heart failure, and interstitial lung disease. DM can be a paraneoplastic disease associated with malignancy in 10% to 20% of patients (31).

A subtype of dermatomyositis known as clinically amyopathic DM (CADM) presents with typical skin changes with minimal or no myopathy. This subtype constitutes 20% of all patients with DM. The anti-CADM-140 antibody has often been found to lead to progressive ILD and can also be used to monitor disease activity in patients with DM and rapidly progressive interstitial lung disease (RP-ILD). CADM is also referred to as skin-predominant dermatomyositis and 'dermatomyositis siné myositis' (DMSM) (32).

Polymyositis (PM)

In polymyositis, the most common clinical presentation is proximal muscle weakness with a subacute onset and significant elevation of the creatinine kinase (CK). It can be difficult to distinguish from other myopathies, and a biopsy plays an important role in distinguishing these entities. Histopathology shows perimysial and endomysial infiltration of macrophages and cytotoxic CD8 T cells.

Necrotizing Myopathy (NM)/ Necrotizing Autoimmune Myopathy (NAM)

This is also known as immune-mediated necrotizing myopathy or necrotizing autoimmune myopathy. There is a progressive, symmetrical proximal muscle weakness of arms and legs. Clinically, it is indistinguishable from PM, and a biopsy is needed to make the diagnosis. It is a heterogenous group of myopathies and includes autoimmune inflammatory mechanisms, paraneoplastic conditions, viral infections (including human immunodeficiency virus and hepatitis C), and exposure to toxins or drugs (most often statins) as well as combinations of these mechanisms. Myositis-specific autoantibodies against single recognition particle (SRP) or 3-hydroxy-3-methylglutaryl co-enzyme A reductase (HMGCR) can be detected in a subset of these patients.

Inclusion Body Myositis (IBM)

IBM is the most frequently acquired myopathy after the fifth decade and is more predominant in males. It is characterized by slow and painless progression over the years and causes asymmetric paresis. The nondominant hand typically gets more severely affected. Flexion of hand, fingers, and knee extension are typically affected. The muscle weakness continues to progress and becomes more generalized over time.

Patients can also develop dysphagia, respiratory muscle weakness, and sleep-disordered breathing requiring nocturnal noninvasive ventilation. The diagnosis often gets delayed until the atrophy is apparent, but early in the disease, weakness is more prominent than atrophy. This subtype of inflammatory muscle disease is often refractory to immunosuppression.

Overlap Syndromes

This group includes patients with myositis who have an underlying connective tissue disease such as systemic lupus erythematosus, rheumatoid arthritis, scleroderma, or mixed connective tissue disease. These are associated with autoantibodies such as Jo-1, PM/SCL, U1RNP, and others.

This group also includes antisynthetase syndrome. Symptoms commonly associated with this syndrome include muscle weakness, inflammatory arthritis, fever, Raynaud's phenomenon, interstitial lung disease, and mechanic's hands. Eight antisynthetase antibodies have been identified as being significant in antisynthetase syndrome myositis, out of which Jo-1 antibody is the most common. Others include PL-7 and PL-12. The remaining five antibodies are much rarer, and their implications are not well understood yet.

MYOSITIS-SPECIFIC AUTOANTIBODIES (MSA) AND ASSOCIATED DISEASES

These antibodies can provide an insight about prognosis and further characterize different classes of myositis. For instance, anti-TIF1-γ antibody (human transcriptional intermediary factor) and anti-NXP2 antibodies can be associated with cancer, which is not likely in Jo-1 antibody positive myositis. Table 7.3 provides a summary of myositis specific and myositis associated antibodies.

Pathogenesis

In dermatomyositis, the binding of immune complexes to endothelial cells causes subsequent activation of the complement pathway and cell lysis mediated by membrane attack complex (MAC).

Table 7.3 Myosotis Specific and Myositis-Associated Antibodies

Antibodies	Association with myositis
Jo 1	—Antisynthetase syndrome
	—PM
	—DM
	—ILD
PL-7, PL-12, OJ, EJ, KS, Ha, and Zo	—Antisynthetase syndrome
Anti–signal recognition particle (SRP)	—Necrotizing myopathy
Anti-TIF1-γ antibody (human transcriptional intermediary factor)	—Children: juvenile dermatomyositis
	—Adults: dermatomyositis
	—Increased risk of cancer-associated DM
Anti-NXP2 (nuclear matrix protein 2)	—DM
	—Increased risk of cancer
	—Increased risk of calcinosis
Anti-SAE (anti–small ubiquitin like modifier activating enzyme heterodimer)	—DM associated with dysphagia and severe skin disease
	—Increased risk of cancer in dermatomyositis
IFN-induced melanoma differentiation-associated protein 5 (MDA5)	—DM, mainly DMSM or CADM
	—Rapidly progressive ILD in children and adults
anti-CADM-140	—Rapid progressive ILD
Anti-PM/Scl	—ILD
	—Overlap of polymyositis and scleroderma
	—Children with PM-scleroderma overlap tend to have a strongly positive antinuclear antibody (ANA)
HMGCR (3-hydroxy-3-methylglutaryl-coenzyme A reductase)	-Statin-induced necrotizing myopathy even in cases when statins were never taken
Anti-Ro/SSA antibody	-Most prevalent myositis-associated autoantibodies (MAA) in myositis
	—Frequently occurs together with anti-ARS antibodies or other MAAs
Mi2	—DM
SUMO-1-activating enzyme heterodimer (SAE)	—DM
Anti 155/140 antibody	—Strong association with malignancy

This leads to cell necrosis and reduces the number of capillaries in muscles. This affects the blood supply and causes perifascicular atrophy. The skin manifestations are due to vacuolar degeneration of epidermal basal cells with epidermal atrophy and dermatitis with lymphocytes and macrophages.

The pathogenesis of polymyositis is characterized by local immune cell activation in skeletal muscles. Expression of proinflammatory cytokines like IFN-γ, IL-6, IL-1β, tumor necrosis factor (TNF)-α, and TGF-β, as well as chemokines such as IL-8, CCL-2, CCL-3, CCL-4, CCL-5, CXCL-9, and CXCL-10, contribute to local inflammation.

Necrotizing myopathy constitutes of a heterogenous group and includes autoimmune inflammatory mechanisms, paraneoplastic conditions, exposure to toxins or drugs, and combinations of these mechanisms. Statins and fibrates are well established to cause toxic myopathy, and the risk increases with an increase in daily dosage of statin. Two-thirds of inflammatory myositis patients with HMGCR autoantibodies have previously been exposed to statins.

Inclusion body myositis has inflammatory changes similar to polymyositis and degenerative changes. There is invasion by macrophages and cytotoxic CD8 T cells with overexpression of metalloproteinases 2 and 9. There is impairment of autophagy in patients with IBM, which causes accumulation of degeneration-related proteins, leading to formation of rimmed vacuoles and intracellular deposits of beta amyloid, which can be visualized by Congo red staining (31).

Diagnosis

Diagnosis is based on clinical examination, laboratory values like creatinine kinase levels, autoantibodies, EMG, and biopsy results. Specific patterns of weakness and chronicity may also help differentiate these entities clinically. IBM tends to show involvement of vastus lateralis, sparing rectus femoris. NAM commonly involves the pelvis and adductor muscles, which are relatively spared in DM.

Myositis-specific antibodies play a significant role in further characterizing the types of myositis. EMG often shows small myopathic units, with fibrillation potential.

MRI is also used to assess and identify adequate muscle for biopsy and demonstrate pattern of muscle involvement. It can show edema in the early stages of disease and fatty transformation or muscle atrophy in the later stages. Fascial and subcutaneous edema is characteristic of DM, although if occurring in dependent areas, disuse and other noninflammatory conditions should be considered in the differential.

Muscle biopsy is the most invasive but definitive step in diagnosis. Although due to the patchy nature of some myositis (patchy involvement can occur in DM), nearly 23% of patients can have false negative biopsies, but it is still considered the gold standard for IIM diagnosis. Necrotizing myopathy is clinically indistinguishable from polymyositis, and a biopsy is required to make the diagnosis. It shows scattered necrotic fibers and macrophage-predominant inflammatory cells. The 2017 EULAR/ACR classification criteria also utilize biopsy finding to calculate the score needed to make the diagnosis of myositis.

Obtaining baseline EKG, echocardiogram, and pulmonary function tests is also recommended in these patients. Patients with suspicion of ILD should have an HRCT, and when dysphagia is reported, video fluoroscopy or flexible endoscopic evaluation of swallowing (FEES) is performed. Patients suffering from subtypes of IIM known to be associated with higher incidence of malignancy should be up to date with age-appropriate cancer screening tests (31, 33).

Management

Glucocorticoid therapy is considered a first-line treatment in patients with myositis. Dosing is usually initiated at 1 mg/kg dosing for 4 to 8 weeks. After disease stabilization, it is slowly weaned, depending on clinical response and side effects. In rapidly progressive cases, with severe weakness or respiratory failure, treatment is usually initiated with pulsed intravenous glucocorticoids, for example, 250 to 1000 mg prednisolone per day for 3 to 5 days.

Mild to moderate disease may be successfully treated with the addition of steroid-sparing agents like methotrexate (MTX), azathioprine, or mycophenolate. MTX is usually started as a 10 to 15 milligrams weekly dose. Azathioprine is started at a daily dosage of 50 mg daily for a week followed by weekly dosage increase if needed. Mycophenolate can also be used at a dose of 500 mg twice daily and can be increased to 2 to 3 gm daily. Combination therapy is not unusual in refractory cases.

Patients with aggressive disease require induction therapy with high-dose IVIG given monthly. Tapering depends upon the treatment effect. Alternatively, rituximab (1 g given on two occasions, 2 weeks apart) may be considered for induction treatment in selected patients.

Treatment response is monitored clinically and by serial serum creatinine kinase (CK) levels. They are a useful marker to assess treatment response and relapse. CK starts to fall prior to any clinically detectable improvement in strength, and elevated levels usually precede clinical relapse. Worsening weakness in spite of a CK level that is improving should trigger consideration of steroid-induced myopathy.

A multidisciplinary team of providers is needed that includes physiotherapist, occupational therapist, and speech therapist to provide exercise programs, fall prevention, and home assessments as well as safe swallowing strategies and nutritional support.

There have been small studies and case series in which biologics like tocilizumab, abatacept, sifalimumab, and tofacitinib were successfully deployed, but more detailed studies are needed

Gastrointestinal Manifestations of Myositis

Distal esophageal dysmotility is by far the most common GI complication in myositis and has been reported in up to two-thirds of adults with dermatomyositis. Delayed gastric emptying and dysmotility are also sometimes seen. However, additional involvement of the gastrointestinal (GI) tract in myositis is rare (in contrast to SSc). One life-threatening manifestation is bowel ischemia as a result of vasculitis or other microvascular processes and is most frequently seen in juvenile dermatomyositis. Vascular injury also likely underpins the rarer findings of gastrointestinal ulceration, hemorrhage, perforation, or intestinal pneumatosis (34). Radiological features typically observed in these cases include widespread thickening of mucosal folds and 'stacked coin' appearance of the small intestine (35). The clinical presentation includes severe epigastric/abdominal pain, diarrhea, vomiting, oral intolerance, hematemesis, or rectal bleeding. Spontaneous bowel perforation or complicated ulcers should be suspected in particularly sick patients.

CONCLUSION

Although the involvement of the GI tract in myositis remains rare, it is important to recognize these disease manifestations, as they can lead to significant morbidity and mortality. There is a paucity of data regarding this aspect of the disease, with case reports forming the bulk of the literature. More organized studies are needed to further expand our knowledge of GI disease in inflammatory myopathies.

REFERENCES

1. Rongioletti F, Ferreli C, Atzori L et al. Scleroderma with an update about clinico-pathological correlation. *G Ital Dermatol Venereol.* 2018;153(2):208–15.
2. Fett N. Scleroderma: Nomenclature, etiology, pathogenesis, prognosis, and treatments: Facts and controversies. *Clin Dermatol.* 2013;31(4):432–7.
3. George R, George A, Kumar TS. Update on management of morphea (localized scleroderma) in children. *Indian Dermatol Online J.* 2020;11(2):135–45.
4. Sharma S, Kumar U. Scleroderma overlap syndromes. *Int J Rheum Dis.* 2016;19(9):831–3.
5. Bellando-Randone S, Matucci-Cerinic M. Very early systemic sclerosis and pre-systemic sclerosis: Definition, recognition, clinical relevance and future directions. *Curr Rheumatol Rep.* 2017;19(10):65.
6. Kahaleh MB. The role of vascular endothelium in the pathogenesis of connective tissue disease: Endothelial injury, activation, participation and response. *Clin Exp Rheumatol.* 1990;8(6):595–601.
7. Volkmann ER, Andreasson K, Smith V. Systemic sclerosis. *Lancet.* 2023;401(10373):304–18.
8. Steen VD. Autoantibodies in systemic sclerosis. *Semin Arthritis Rheum.* 2005;35(1):35–42.
9. Kayser C, Fritzler MJ. Autoantibodies in systemic sclerosis: Unanswered questions. *Front Immunol.* 2015;6:167.
10. Ho KT, Reveille JD. The clinical relevance of autoantibodies in scleroderma. *Arthritis Res Ther.* 2003;5(2):80–93.
11. Perelas A, Silver RM, Arrossi AV et al. Systemic sclerosis-associated interstitial lung disease. *Lancet Respir Med.* 2020;8(3):304–20.
12. Deshauer S, Junek M, Baron M et al. Effect of pregnancy on scleroderma progression. *J Scleroderma Relat Disord.* 2023;8(1):27–30.
13. Taraborelli M, Ramoni V, Brucato A et al. Brief report: Successful pregnancies but a higher risk of preterm births in patients with systemic sclerosis: An Italian multicenter study. *Arthritis Rheum.* 2012;64(6):1970–7.
14. Walker AM, Bermas BL, Jacobe HT. Morphea disease activity during pregnancy: A case series. *J Dermatol.* 2022;49(12):1278–83.
15. van den Hoogen F, Khanna D, Fransen J et al. 2013 classification criteria for systemic sclerosis: An American college of rheumatology/European league against rheumatism collaborative initiative. *Arthritis Rheum.* 2013;65(11):2737–47.

16. Khanna D, Lin CJF, Furst DE et al. Long-term safety and efficacy of tocilizumab in early systemic sclerosis-interstitial lung disease: Open-label extension of a phase 3 randomized controlled trial. *Am J Respir Crit Care Med.* 2022;205(6):674–84.

17. Thoua NM, Bunce C, Brough G et al. Assessment of gastrointestinal symptoms in patients with systemic sclerosis in a UK tertiary referral centre. *Rheumatol* (Oxford). 2010;49(9):1770–5.

18. Luquez-Mindiola A, Atuesta AJ, Gomez-Aldana AJ. Gastrointestinal manifestations of systemic sclerosis: An updated review. *World J Clin Cases.* 2021;9(22):6201–17.

19. McFarlane IM, Bhamra MS, Kreps A et al. Gastrointestinal manifestations of systemic sclerosis. *Rheumatol* (Sunnyvale). 2018;8(1).

20. Derk CT, Rasheed M, Spiegel JR et al. Increased incidence of carcinoma of the tongue in patients with systemic sclerosis. *J Rheumatol.* 2005;32(4):637–41.

21. Strek ME. Systemic sclerosis-associated interstitial lung disease: Role of the oesophagus in outcomes. *Respirol.* 2018;23(10):885–6.

22. Selinger CP, Ang YS. Gastric Antral Vascular Ectasia (GAVE): An update on clinical presentation, pathophysiology and treatment. *Digestion.* 2008;77(2):7.

23. Ghrénassia E, Avouac J, Khanna D et al. Prevalence, correlates and outcomes of gastric antral vascular ectasia in systemic sclerosis: A EUSTAR case-control study. *J Rheumatol.* 2014;41(1):7.

24. Kaniecki T, Abdi T, McMahan ZH. A practical approach to the evaluation and management of gastrointestinal symptoms in patients with systemic sclerosis. *Best Pract Res Clin Rheumatol.* 2021;35(3):101666.

25. Campbell PM, LeRoy EC. Pathogenesis of systemic sclerosis: A vascular hypothesis. *Semin Arthritis Rheum.* 1975;4(4):351–68.

26. McMahan ZH, Khanna D. Managing gastrointestinal complications in patients with systemic sclerosis. *Curr Treat Options Gastroenterol.* 2020;18:531–44.

27. Marie I, Ducrotte P, Denis P et al. Small intestinal bacterial overgrowth in systemic sclerosis. *Rheumatol* (Oxford). 2009;48(10):1314–19.

28. Sattar B, Chokshi RV. Colonic and anorectal manifestations of systemic sclerosis. *Curr Gastroenterol Rep.* 2019;21(7):33.

29. Thoua NM, Abdel-Halim M, Forbes A et al. Fecal incontinence in systemic sclerosis is secondary to neuropathy. *Am J Gastroenterol.* 2012;107(4):7.

30. Nagaraja V, McMahan ZH, Getzug T et al. Management of gastrointestinal involvement in scleroderma. *Curr Treatm Opt Rheumatol.* 2015;1(1):82–105.

31. Carstens PO, Schmidt J. Diagnosis, pathogenesis and treatment of myositis: Recent advances. *Clin Exp Immunol.* 2014;175(3):349–58.

32. Sato S, Kuwana M, Fujita T et al. Anti-CADM-140/MDA5 autoantibody titer correlates with disease activity and predicts disease outcome in patients with dermatomyositis and rapidly progressive interstitial lung disease. *Mod Rheumatol.* 2013;23(3):496–502.

33. Moghadam-Kia S, Oddis CV. Current and new targets for treating myositis. *Curr Opin Pharmacol.* 2022;65:102257.

34. Tweezer-Zaks N, Ben-Horin S, Schiby G et al. Severe gastrointestinal inflammation in adult dermatomyositis: Characterization of a novel clinical association. *Am J Med Sci.* 2006 Dec;332(6):308–13.

35. Lin WY, Wang SJ, Hwang DW et al. Technetium-99m-pyrophosphate scintigraphic findings of intestinal perforation in dermatomyositis. *J Nucl Med.* 1995;36(9):1615–17.

8

Vasculitis

ROBERT CORTY, JASON SPRINGER, AND KEVIN BYRAM

INTRODUCTION

Vasculitis describes inflammation of a blood vessel. It becomes clinically significant when the inflammatory process causes either hemodynamically significant luminal narrowing or vessel wall breakdown, either of which can cause tissue ischemia or, when severe, tissue necrosis. Per the 2012 Chapel Hill Consensus Conference Nomenclature of Vasculitides (CHCC), vasculitis syndromes are categorized in to four types: primary vasculitis syndromes (which can be further subdivided based on the predominant size vessel involved), vasculitis associated with systemic auto-immune disease, vasculitis associated with probable etiology, and single-organ vasculitis (1).

The first section of this chapter will discuss primary vasculitis syndromes. In these conditions, evidence of vasculitis is required to confirm the diagnosis, and no cause is known. One of the first primary vasculitis syndromes identified was polyarteritis nodosa (2, 3). Primary vasculitis syndromes are oftentimes difficult to diagnose due to their nonspecific symptoms and the absence of specific, confirmatory lab tests. Thus, either vascular imaging or tissue biopsy is critical to confirm the diagnosis. The second section of this chapter will discuss vasculitides associated with systemic autoimmune diseases (SAID) and other causes. We will describe, for each form of SAID-associated vasculitis, the typical pattern of vascular involvement. One example is lupus-associated mesenteric vasculitis. Other causes of vasculitis syndromes include infection, cancer, and medication exposure. The

third section of this chapter will discuss noninflammatory vascular conditions that can be difficult to distinguish from the vasculitides discussed previously.

In each section, special attention is paid to how the gastrointestinal (GI) manifestations of each form of vasculitis should be suspected, diagnosed, and treated. GI manifestations of systemic vasculitis can be challenging to diagnose for some of the same reasons as vasculitis in general is difficult to diagnose. GI involvement is rare in most forms of vasculitis, and when present, symptoms tend to be nonspecific.

Some overarching concepts apply to all the categories. First, as the final common pathway of disease for all forms of vasculitis is ischemia of the tissue perfused by the affected vasculature, signs and symptoms will manifest based on which vessels are involved. If the mesenteric vasculature is involved, the patient may experience postprandial abdominal pain ("abdominal angina"), nausea, vomiting, diarrhea, and/or hematochezia. Patients with abdominal vasculitis involving the blood supply to the kidneys may experience renovascular hypertension. Patients with microvascular involvement of the mucosa may have ulcers visible on physical exam or endoscopy. Second, the treating clinician must consider a broad differential diagnosis including nonvasculitis mimics (e.g., Ehlers-Danlos syndrome, thromboembolic disease, infections, etc.). Third, whenever GI vasculitis is suspected or diagnosed, the treating physician should consider consultation with a rheumatologist. Accurate diagnosis of the underlying cause of

DOI: 10.1201/9781003367307-8

GI pathology may depend on elicitation of extra-GI symptoms to identify a systemic disease. For example, a patient presenting with abdominal pain and a headache, once found to have vasculitis of the mesenteric arteries, should undergo imaging of the cranial vasculature as part of an evaluation for polyarteritis nodosa.

By reading this chapter, the reader will develop knowledge on the diagnosis and management of GI manifestations of (1) common primary systemic vasculitis syndromes, (2) vasculitides secondary to SAIDs and other causes, and (3) noninflammatory mimics of vasculitis.

PRIMARY SYSTEMIC VASCULITIDES

IgA Vasculitis

DEFINITION

According to the 2012 CHCC, IgA vasculitis is a small-vessel vasculitis characterized by pathogenic IgA1 deposits in affected tissues, often with associated cutaneous involvement (classically palpable purpura), GI involvement, and joint pain. This disease was formerly known as Henoch-Schönlein purpura and was renamed in 2012 in recognition of the pathologic role of abnormal IgA1 in serum and its deposition in affected vessels (1).

CLASSIFICATION/DIAGNOSTIC CRITERIA

For children, the most recent set of classification criteria comes from the 2008 Ankara Consensus Conference. A patient meets these criteria when they have lower-limb predominant purpura not related to thrombocytopenia plus one of the following four: (1) abdominal pain, (2) histopathologic evidence, typically leukocytoclastic vasculitis with predominant IgA deposits, (3) acute arthralgias, or (4) renal involvement such as proteinuria, hematuria, or red blood cell casts in urine sediment (4).

For adults, the most recent set of classification criteria is the American College of Rheumatology (ACR) 1990 Criteria for the Classification of Henoch-Schönlein Purpura. Patients meet these criteria with two of the following four: (1) palpable purpura without thrombocytopenia, (2) age less than 20 years at disease onset, (3) bowel angina, which can manifest with abdominal pain worse after meals or other evidence of bowel ischemia

such as bloody diarrhea, and (4) granulocytes in the walls of arterioles or venules seen on histologic exam (5). It is important to understand that established classification criteria like these do not have perfect sensitivity or specificity for the diagnosis of disease. Patients of all ages can develop IgA vasculitis.

There are no diagnostic criteria validated for clinical use.

EPIDEMIOLOGY

IgA vasculitis is the most common form of vasculitis in children and is relatively rare in adults. Most cases of IgA vasculitis occur in children under the age of 12. The annual incidence among children ranges from 6 to 30 per 100,000 patient-years, with peak incidence in the age range of 4 to 9. There is an almost even distribution by gender (1–1.5:1 male-to-female ratio). More cases are diagnosed in winter (1.5:1 ratio of winter to summer presentations) (6–10). Few studies offer a specific incidence among adults, perhaps due to its rarity; but estimates are generally in the range of 1 to 5 per 100,00 patient-years, with an average age at diagnosis of 50 to 60 years (11, 12).

GASTROINTESTINAL MANIFESTATIONS

GI manifestations in IgA vasculitis are fairly common in both children and adults. One of the most feared GI complications in IgA vasculitis is intussusception and resulting bowel ischemia. This complication is rare in adults but more common in children. Among adults, gastrointestinal manifestations in general are less common but more severe. Gastrointestinal manifestations of IgA vasculitis were recently reported by the French Vasculitis Study Group (13, 14). Among this cohort of 260 adult patients, 53% had gastrointestinal involvement. Of those with gastrointestinal involvement, all had abdominal pain, 31% intestinal bleeding, 26% diarrhea, 19% nausea or emesis, 9% paralytic ileus, and 4% required abdominal surgery. On imaging and endoscopic evaluation, 61% had thickening of the intestinal wall, and 87% had endoscopic abnormalities, predominantly mucosal ulcerations but also including mucosal erythema and purpura. Inflammatory infiltrate on histology was seen in half (3/6) of patients with endoscopic stomach biopsies and all (8/8) with endoscopic intestinal biopsies. Patients with gastrointestinal involvement were slightly younger, constitutionally sicker, more likely to have arthralgias, and had slightly higher C-reactive protein levels (3.7 vs. 1.9 mg/dL) than patients without gastrointestinal involvement. Patients with gastrointestinal involvement had a similar clinical response rate (40% to 50%) and relapse rate (10% to 15%) as patients without gastrointestinal involvement. Two patients with gastrointestinal involvement died from IgA vasculitis-related causes: one from septic shock due to gastrointestinal perforation due to ischemia after 1 month on glucocorticoid therapy and the other from acute renal injury and mesenteric ischemia after 3 months on glucocorticoid therapy.

One prospective study of adults with biopsy-proven IgA vasculitis found that about half have GI involvement as defined simply by the presence of abdominal pain, and half of this subgroup had severe involvement as defined by gastrointestinal hemorrhage or bowel ischemia (15). A small study that was enriched for patients with relapsing disease noted that 80% have gastrointestinal involvement, 40% with gastrointestinal hemorrhage (16).

TREATMENT

Among children, most cases are mild and self-limited (17). For such cases, which are characterized by lower extremity purpura, joint pains, abdominal pain without evidence of massive gastrointestinal bleeding or perforation, and mild or no kidney involvement, symptomatic treatment is appropriate including NSAID therapy with consideration of colchicine. For more severe gastrointestinal manifestations, as described earlier, high-dose glucocorticoids are the mainstay of therapy (18). Mycophenolate mofetil, azathioprine, and cyclophosphamide are recommended by consensus guidelines for moderate to severe renal manifestations, though only low-quality evidence supports these recommendations (18).

In adults, treatment for IgA vasculitis is targeted toward specific manifestations, and high-level evidence is generally lacking, especially for severe manifestations. Patients with joint pains should be treated with pharmacologic pain control as needed. Patients with abdominal pain without severe GI involvement should be managed with antispasmodics, avoidance of large meals, and pain management. Severe GI involvement, as defined by massive bleeding, peritonitis, or radiologic evidence of perforation, should be evaluated surgically and considered for intravenous methylprednisolone and a three-month course of oral prednisone starting at approximately 1 mg/kg (19). One can consider the addition of cyclophosphamide for severe cases, though the one small, randomized controlled trial examining its addition to glucocorticoids found no difference in outcome between arms (15). Interestingly, one retrospective analysis that used statistical corrections for disease severity suggested cyclophosphamide may be beneficial when added to glucocorticoids (14). One observation study of 22 patients with refractory or relapsed IgA vasculitis found that clinical outcomes tended to be good after rituximab therapy (16).

If high-dose glucocorticoids are used in a patient with abdominal involvement of IgA vasculitis, the clinician should remain highly sensitive to clinical decline with respect to the abdomen. High-dose glucocorticoids can blunt the sensitivity of a physical exam for gastrointestinal perforation. Fever curve, trajectory of inflammatory markers, and serial imaging should be used to monitor such a patient for clinical change.

Renal involvement is a separate indication for immunosuppression. However, the details of decision-making driven by renal involvement are outside the scope of this chapter.

Polyarteritis Nodosa and Related Conditions

DEFINITION

Polyarteritis nodosa (PAN) was one of the first vasculitis syndromes to be reported in the medical literature, though it was originally termed "periarteritis nodosa" (3). Today, PAN is understood to be a vasculitis syndrome that affects small to medium arteries, with a predilection for medium arteries, characterized by histological evidence of vessel wall necrosis, absence of glomerulonephritis, and absence of antineutrophil cytoplasmic antibodies (ANCAs) (1). The absence of glomerulonephritis and ANCA serologies serves to distinguish PAN from forms of ANCA-associated vasculitis, such as microscopic polyangiitis (MPA), a distinction not formally made prior to the 1994 Chapel Hill Consensus Conference (20). As opposed to MPA, PAN is characterized by the absence of arteriole or end capillary involvement. Thus, older historical

PAN cohort studies must now be viewed critically as possibly containing patients with ANCA-associated vasculitides, primarily MPA (5, 20). Furthermore, in 1970, the strong association between hepatitis B and PAN was first described (21). As of the 2012 CHCC, PAN associated with hepatitis B was redefined as "HBV-associated vasculitis," not primary PAN (1, 22). Modern genetic approaches to diagnostics have shown evidence that monogenic variants can cause syndromes that appear clinically similar to PAN (e.g., adenosine deaminase 2 syndrome), and the existence of such syndromes is not yet reflected in any systemic classification criteria. Thus, the prevalence of primary PAN has significantly declined as secondary causes with PAN-like presentations have been discovered. Here, we discuss primary PAN, infection-associated medium-vessel vasculitis, and conditions similar to PAN that are attributable to monogenic variants.

EPIDEMIOLOGY

Considering the complexity in naming and categorizing PAN and related conditions as well as their rarity, incidence is challenging to estimate. The most recent estimate comes from a retrospective chart review in Poland for the years 2008–2013, which estimated an incidence of 2.4 cases per million person-years, with a trend downward from 3.3 at the start of the study period to 1.9 at the end of the study period (23). Prior estimates are in the range of 6.2 to 9.7 cases per million person-years, with a slight male predominance (1–1.5:1 male:female), and a typical age of onset in the 40s to 70s (24, 25). In light of repeated changes in classification, earlier studies should be interpreted to have an additional layer of uncertainty.

GASTROINTESTINAL MANIFESTATIONS

The most common manifestations of PAN are constitutional, neurologic, renal, and cutaneous. PAN should be considered in a patient with fever of unknown origin, new-onset renovascular hypertension, mononeuritis multiplex, or medium-vessel phenomena in the skin, like tender painful nodules or livedo racemosa. However, gastrointestinal involvement is important to recognize since it can be severe and has been associated with a poor prognosis, especially when requiring surgery (26, 27). Approximately 40% of patients have gastrointestinal manifestations, most commonly

abdominal pain. Approximately 10% of patients have severe enough abdominal pain or GI hemorrhage to warrant abdominal surgery (27). The most common imaging findings in these severe cases are fusiform stenosis and microaneurysms of the mesenteric, renal, or hepatic arteries. It is important to note that the microaneurysms of PAN may be below the resolution of CTA or MRA and better visualized by traditional catheter-based angiography, although these imaging techniques are continually evolving in their precision. In cases in which abdominal surgery is required for therapeutic purposes, intestinal tissue may be available for sampling to confirm diagnosis with demonstration of a medium-vessel vasculitis (Figure 8.1).

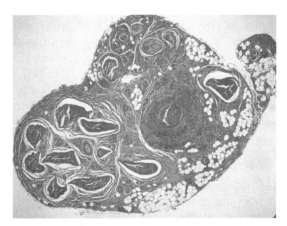

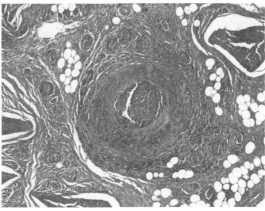

Figure 8.1 Representative histology of vasa nervorum of the sural nerve of a patient with polyarteritis nodosa. This 19-year-old man presented to care for fever of unknown origin, weight loss, mononeuritis, vague abdominal pain, and tender skin nodules. Note the transmural inflammatory infiltrate, extravasated red blood cells, and fibrinoid necrosis.

TREATMENT

For patients diagnosed with classic PAN that is not severe (i.e., immediately life- or organ-threatening), the American College of Rheumatology/Vasculitis Foundation guidelines recommend treatment with glucocorticoids and a conventional synthetic DMARD such as azathioprine or methotrexate. For patients with severe PAN, the same guideline recommends treatment with glucocorticoids and cyclophosphamide (28).

POLYARTERITIS NODOSA SECONDARY TO INFECTION OR MEDICATION

Epidemiology

The incidence of HBV-associated PAN, also known as HBV-associated vasculitis, is directly proportional to HBV infection rates. With widespread vaccination available, its incidence has dropped precipitously in the developed world, where it is now very rare. PAN associated with HIV and HCV has also been reported but are uncommon (29, 30). Rare cases of medication-induced PAN have been described, with minocycline the most frequently implicated medication (31).

Gastrointestinal Manifestations

As with classic PAN, the most frequent manifestations are constitutional, neurologic, and renal. However, cutaneous manifestations are modestly less likely in HBV-PAN (35% vs. 57%), and GI symptoms are slightly more common (50% vs. 30%). Up to 72% of patients with HBV-PAN have angiographic evidence of mesenteric involvement, compared to only 49% of patients with classic PAN (27). Patients with HBV-PAN have a higher risk of requiring abdominal surgery when compared to patients with classic PAN (20% vs. 10%). No unique or specific patterns of symptoms have been reported for HCV-associated PAN or HIV-associated PAN.

Treatment

Patients with HBV-PAN that is not severe (i.e., not organ- or life-threatening) can be treated by directly treating the HBV infection in consultation with an infectious disease or hepatology specialist. For patients with severe disease, high-quality evidence is lacking. Treatment of the underlying HBV infection should remain the mainstay of therapy, but sometimes, immunosuppressives are essential to treat tissue-level inflammatory activity to prevent irreversible damage. In these instances, strong consideration should be given to glucocorticoids at high dose (e.g., 1 mg/kg for one week and tapering over several weeks). Another therapy that has been documented to improve outcomes, though without randomized evidence, is plasma exchange (32).

POLYARTERITIS NODOSA-LIKE SYNDROME DUE TO MONOGENIC VARIANT

Familial Mediterranean Fever

Familial Mediterranean fever (FMF) is a monogenic disease caused by an inherited mutation in the *MEFV* gene, which encodes *pyrin* (33). It is common in the Middle East with a prevalence of 250 to 1,000 per 100,000 persons in Turkey, 1,000 per 100,000 persons in Israel, and 500 per 100,000 persons in Armenia, and rare in populations without genetic inheritance from the Middle East (34–37). Mutations in *pyrin* lead to inappropriate IL1β expression, which manifests with recurrent episodes of fever, serositis, and rash, with asymptomatic periods in between, though there is variation according to the specific variant in MEFV (38). Treatment with colchicine is usually sufficient to prevent attacks, but for cases resistant to colchicine therapy, IL1β inhibition with canakinumab is typically effective (39). If undertreated, however, patients can develop amyloidosis, small bowel obstruction, or vasculitis reminiscent of primary PAN or IgA vasculitis (40, 41). Case series have reported successful treatment of FMF-associated medium-vessel vasculitis, with glucocorticoids and/or IL1β inhibitor therapy (41).

Deficiency of Adenosine Deaminase 2

Deficiency of adenosine deaminase 2 (DADA2) is a monogenic disease caused by an inherited, loss-of-function mutation in the *CER1* gene, which encodes ADA2, a driver of macrophage differentiation, toward an anti-inflammatory phenotype (42, 43). Patients typically present in the first decade of life, though onset in adulthood has been reported due to varied penetrance. Patients will manifest with features of medium-vessel vasculitis, including nodular cutaneous disease, abdominal vasculitis, and stroke, with additional features of immunodeficiency such as frequent or opportunistic infections. Sequencing-based screening approaches have revealed up to 7% of patients with classic PAN might actually have DADA2 (44). TNF inhibitors have been shown to decrease substantially the risk of stroke in these patients (45).

Behçet Disease

DEFINITION

Behçet disease is a rare, variable-vessel vasculitis that usually manifests initially with recurrent oral and genital ulcers and is often associated with inflammatory lesions of the eye, joints, gastrointestinal tract, and central nervous system. Unique among the primary systemic vasculitides, it often prominently involves thrombosis in addition to vasculitis (including both arteritis and venulitis) (1).

EPIDEMIOLOGY

Behçet disease affects men and women with equal frequency and has wide geographic variation in incidence and prevalence (46). It typically has onset in the third or fourth decade of life (46). Incidence is estimated at 0.2 per 100,000 person-years in Sweden and 0.4 per 100,000 person-years in the United States (47, 48). A complex interplay of genetics and environmental factors leads to such regional prevalence estimates as disparate as less than 1 per 100,000 in the United Kingdom to 370 per 100,000 in Turkey. Interestingly, persons with Turkish ancestry living in Germany have a prevalence of Behçet disease of 77 per 100,000, in between the rate of those who live in Turkey (370) and Germans of German ancestry (1.5) (46).

PATHOPHYSIOLOGY

The precise cause and pathophysiology of Behçet disease is not fully understood, but it has both genetic and environmental contributions. The strongest genetic risk factor is HLA-B*51 (49). Additionally, mutations in *ERAP1*, which is important in processing of peptides that will be displayed by T cells, as well as IL17F and IL23A, have been found to predispose toward Behçet disease (46). The causative environmental factors are unknown. The effector cells in Behçet disease include excessive Th1 activation mediated by IL-12 and IL-10 as well as neutrophils activated by Th17 cells in the presence of IL-23.

DIAGNOSIS

The most commonly cited diagnostic criteria for Behçet disease are the 1990 International Study Group (ISG) for Behçet disease: recurrent oral ulcers plus two of the following four findings—(1) recurrent genital ulcers, (2) eye lesions consistent with Behçet disease, (3) skin lesions consistent with Behçet disease, and (4) a positive pathergy test (50). These criteria have two primary limitations. First, the cohort in which they were derived contained 80% Middle Eastern, patients and the disease manifestations vary across genetic backgrounds. Most notable here is the relative rarity of GI manifestations among Middle Eastern patients as compared to patients with Western or East Asian genetic background (51). The second limitation is that the control cohort did not include patients with inflammatory bowel diseases, which are often the most clinically challenging conditions to distinguish from Behçet disease (46). A third limitation, inherent to any set of criteria applied internationally, is that the base rates of the components of the score and the various competing diagnosis is different across geographies, so the performance of the diagnostic criteria is inconsistent.

These limitations led to the collaborative work across 27 countries to develop the International Criteria for Behçet Disease (ICBD) (52). What these criteria gain in international applicability, they lose in specificity, with specificity of 90% as compared to 95% for the ISG criteria (52). Fortunately, the ICBD criteria also include an interpretation of the probability of Behçet disease for each point total, ranging from "almost certainly not BD" to "almost certainly BD" rather than a simple binary cutoff, so a clinician can tailor their use to the sensitivity and specificity demands of the clinical scenario.

Behçet disease should be considered in a patient with recurrent oral and genital ulcers, with other typical manifestations of BD, including uveitis, retinal vasculitis, venous or arterial thrombosis, or neurologic syndromes. Patients with BD can present with inflammatory oligoarthritis. Patients with BD can have a variety of cutaneous manifestations, including pyoderma gangrenosum-like lesions, pustular acneiform lesions, or nodular panniculitic lesions resembling erythema nodosum.

GASTROINTESTINAL MANIFESTATIONS

Almost all patients with Behçet disease have ulcers in the mouth (46, 51). These lesions are typically small, with approximately one new lesion per week, and each lasting an average of 1 week. Multiple lesions can exist at one time, and they may be exquisitely painful and distressing in severe cases.

The largest Behçet disease cohort consists of 387 patients with an average of 20 years' disease duration in Istanbul, Turkey. None of these patients were reported to have gastrointestinal involvement, and population estimates suggest 1% to 3% of Middle Eastern patients with BD will develop intestinal complications (46, 53).

By contrast, the frequency of intestinal gastrointestinal involvement in East Asian patients is 5% to 25% (46). Patients most commonly have diarrhea, abdominal pain, gastrointestinal bleeding, or weight loss but can have one or a few large, deep intestinal ulcers seen on endoscopy. They are commonly near the ileocecal junction and have onset about 5 years after diagnosis (54, 55). Five percent to 10% of patients have ulceration of the esophagus, stomach, or duodenum, and a further 20% to 30% have ulceration of the colon (56). The manifestations in Behçet disease can closely mimic inflammatory bowel disease, but the presence of scarring genital ulceration should prompt the clinician to consider Behçet disease as the more likely diagnosis.

A large, retrospective analysis of patients with BD found that approximately 15% had vascular involvement (57). The majority of these patients (67%) had DVT only, while an additional 20% had DVT alongside another vascular thrombotic event. Ten percent of patients had pulmonary embolism. Six percent of patients had an extrapulmonary arterial event, which could include portal and mesenteric arteritis but could also include cerebral, retinal, coronary, or renal disease. Figure 8.2 shows one such rare case of a celiac artery aneurysm. BD has a classic association with Budd–Chiari syndrome (thrombosis of the hepatic vein), though this is empirically rare and found in only 2% of cases.

MANAGEMENT

For mucocutaneous lesions, topical steroids are the first line. Colchicine should be used to prevent recurrence (58). Apremilast has also been shown to be effective in improving the number of oral ulcers and the associated pain in Behçet disease (59). For

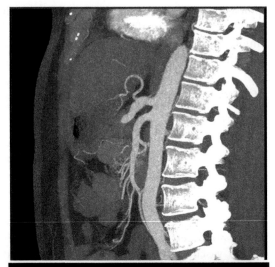
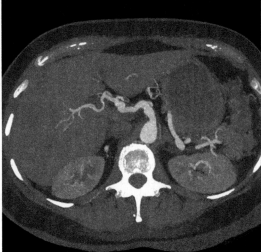
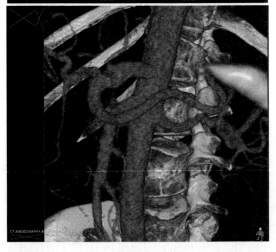

Figure 8.2 CTA of a middle-aged woman with Behçet disease. Celiac artery shows aneurysmal irregularity.

patients who fail these standard therapies, TNF inhibitors can be considered (58, 60, 61).

For patients with BD with any signs or symptoms suggestive of gastrointestinal involvement, physicians should obtain cross-sectional imaging and/or endoscopic studies to determine the extent and location of disease.

Pulmonary artery aneurysm is a major cause of mortality in patients with BD, so it should be screened for at diagnosis in all patients and revisited if the patient develops any suspicious such as new iron deficiency anemia, dyspnea, or hemoptysis. Patients with other vascular findings such as DVT or dural sinus thrombosis are at higher risk of this rare but often fatal finding.

During an acute flare that involves gastro-intestinal ulcers, glucocorticoid therapy should be used, and surgical consultation should be sought when there is concern for perforation, major bleeding, or obstruction (58). Per updated consensus guidelines, chronic management of GI involvement should involve 5-ASA or azathioprine with potential recourse to TNF inhibitors or, in the most resistant cases, thalidomide (58).

Giant Cell Arteritis

DEFINITION AND DIAGNOSIS

Giant cell arteritis (GCA) refers to a primary systemic vasculitis syndrome that almost exclusively occurs among patients over age 50. It predominantly affects the aorta and its major branches, often branches off the carotid and vertebral arteries such as the temporal artery, and often has granulomatous inflammation (1).

EPIDEMIOLOGY

Selecting for the population of age greater than 50 years, the incidence and prevalence of GCA have been estimated at 10 cases per 100,000 person-years and 51 cases per 100,000 people (62). It is reported to have higher incidence at higher latitudes as compared to lower latitudes (62). Historically, clinicians have considered GCA to be more prevalent in patients of European and Scandinavian descent, but recent analyses have shown about equal prevalence in various populations including Black patients (63).

MANIFESTATIONS

A typical case of GCA involves a patient in the seventh decade of life or older with a few weeks of malaise and weight loss who presents to clinic with new-onset, lateral headache, with scalp tenderness on the same side, possibly sudden vision loss, and is found to have elevated sedimentation rate and C-reactive protein. Some patients have associated aortitis (64). In cases of cranial involvement, temporal artery biopsy is the gold standard for confirming the diagnosis. In other cases, imaging studies such as temporal artery ultrasound, CT angiography, and even FDG-PET may reveal areas of arterial stenosis and/or inflammation. GI manifestations of GCA are rare. In two of the largest cohorts, GCA has been reported to affect the mesentery in 1% and 22% of patients, a wide disparity (65). Previously, a pooled analysis of the two other tertiary referral center GCA cohorts indicated that the mesenteric artery is involved in 18% of patients (66). Though it is rare, there are case reports of GCA affecting the tongue, even causing necrosis, presumably due to ischemic involvement of the lingual artery (67, 68).

MANAGEMENT

Current guidelines recommend treatment of most patients with GCA with a glucocorticoid course and tocilizumab, an inhibitor of interleukin-6 (69). From a GI perspective, one potential toxicity to consider from tocilizumab is the increased risk for development of diverticulitis and gastrointestinal perforation that has been seen in the RA population in some postmarketing studies but not in others (70, 71). This toxicity was not observed in the long-term follow-up of the largest RCT on GCA. However, patients with a history of diverticulitis were excluded, and the small sample size limits detection of rare adverse events (72).

Takayasu Arteritis

DEFINITION

Takayasu arteritis (TAK) is a systemic vasculitis syndrome characterized by inflammation of the aorta and its branches, typically granulomatous on histological examination, that affects patients younger than age 50 and more commonly affects women than men (1).

EPIDEMIOLOGY

TAK is a rare disease with an incidence rate estimated by meta-analysis to be approximately one case per million person-years. It is more common among women, with around two cases per million years, and there is marked heterogeneity among studied analysed (73). The rate may be higher in Asian populations, where the disease was originally described, with one study in Korea estimating an incidence of 2 cases per million person-years and prevalence of 28 cases per million persons (74).

MANIFESTATIONS

The most common symptoms at the time of diagnosis are constitutional and cardiovascular. Up to 80% of patients have constitutional symptoms such as fever, fatigue, malaise, weight loss, or night sweats (75). Eighty percent of patients have cardiovascular symptoms such as tachycardia, palpitations, renovascular hypertension, upper limb claudication, carotidynia, or upper extremity pulse discrepancy. Gastrointestinal symptoms are less common, with approximately 10% of patients having abdominal pain, nausea, vomiting, or diarrhea, suspicious for proximal mesenteric and/ or celiac artery involvement. However, on angiographic imaging, 30% of patients have involvement of the mesenteric arteries, with an equal division between superior and inferior mesenteric arteries (65, 76, 77). Typically, patients will not have symptoms unless multiple mesenteric/celiac arteries are involved. Approximately 75% of the mesenteric lesions are stenotic, with the remainder demonstrating complete occlusion (76). The most severe gastrointestinal complication is bowel ischemia requiring surgical intervention. In one study of 60 patients, 1 patient had dissection of the superior mesenteric artery (77). One study of 105 patients in Canada noted that 4% had bowel ischemia, a figure that rose to 13% in patients who fit in the aortic-renal-gastric involvement disease cluster (78). In another study of 126 patients in the United States, 4% of patients had mesenteric ischemia (76). A retrospective study of 318 patients in France reported that of the 16 patients who died, 3 died from complications of mesenteric ischemia, though the number of patients who suffered from this problem and survived was not reported (79).

MANAGEMENT

Upon diagnosis of active disease, glucocorticoids are the mainstay of initial treatment, with dosage corresponding to disease severity. For manifestations that are immediately life- or organ-threatening, intravenous "pulse" doses of methylprednisolone, 250 mg or greater over 1 to 5 days, may be appropriate. For severe disease that does not fit the listed characteristics, approximately 1 mg per kg is appropriate, and for moderate disease, 0.5 mg per kg is appropriate. In all cases, a long taper to low-dose prednisone ($\leq$ 10 mg/d or equivalent) is appropriate. With approximately 40% of patients experiencing disease recurrence in the 10 years after diagnosis and unacceptable toxicity from long-term, high-dose steroid use, a steroid-sparing agent is typically added soon after diagnosis. Conventional DMARDs in common use include methotrexate and azathioprine, though the evidence supporting these is of low quality (80). The most common biologics in use for management of TAK are TNF inhibitors, though the level of evidence is also low (81). Two small randomized controlled trials examined tocilizumab, an IL6 inhibitor, and abatacept, a CTLA4 inhibitor, in addition to glucocorticoids, and neither found superiority compared to glucocorticoids alone, though their power was low (82, 83). A study of patients with TAK in China found tofacitinib, a JAK inhibitor, to be superior to methotrexate as a steroid-sparing agent (84).

ANCA-Associated Vasculitides

Antineutrophil cytoplasmic antibody (ANCA)-associated vasculitis (AAV) refers to three primary vasculitis syndromes that cause vascular necrosis, predominantly in arterioles, capillaries, and venules. Most patients have a positive ANCA test (~90%). The three types of AAV are microscopic polyangiitis (MPA), granulomatosis with polyangiitis (GPA), and eosinophilic granulomatosis with polyangiitis (eGPA) (1). At the time of publication, there is an ongoing debate as to the most clinically useful way to classify AAVs between the traditional phenotype-based classification and the relatively novel antibody-based classification or some combination of the two (85). Some cases of MPA and GPA have been attributed to medications. Hydralazine, propylthiouracil, methimazole, minocycline, cocaine, and levamisole are the most frequently cited medications associated with AAV (86, 87).

DEFINITIONS

Microscopic polyangiitis (MPA) causes necrotizing, nongranulomatous, pauci-immune vasculitis that predominantly affects small and sometimes medium sized arteries. The most commonly involved organs are the skin, kidney, and lung, with glomerulonephritis and pulmonary capillaritis being particularly devastating manifestations. Almost all patients will have positive ANCA testing, most commonly with antibodies to both myeloperoxidase on ELISA testing and perinuclear staining (p-ANCA) on immunofluorescence (88). Granulomatosis with polyangiitis (GPA) is a necrotizing, granulomatous systemic vasculitis that predominantly affects small vessels and sometimes medium arteries and veins, with a predilection for the kidneys (glomerulonephritis). It is known to favor the upper respiratory tract and sinuses as well (89). Of patients with GPA, approximately 75% have a positive PR3-ANCA test, while 15% have a positive MPO-ANCA test and 10% are ANCA-negative (90). Eosinophilic granulomatosis with polyangiitis (EGPA) is similar to GPA in that it causes granulomatous inflammation and necrotizing vasculitis of small and medium vessels but differs in that the inflammatory infiltrate has a profound eosinophilia, the peripheral eosinophil count is usually elevated, and adult-onset asthma is characteristic.

EPIDEMIOLOGY

MPA is a rare disease with incidence between 2.7 and 14 cases per million person-years and prevalence between 9 and 184 cases per million adults (91). GPA is similarly rare with incidence between 3 and 13 cases per million person-years and prevalence between 23 and 218 cases per million adults (91). EGPA is yet rarer with incidence between 0.5 and 4 cases per million person-years and prevalence between 2 and 22 cases per million adults (91).

GI MANIFESTATIONS

The FVSG cohort is the largest assembled for study of ANCA-associated vasculitides. In the FVSG cohort, approximately 16% of patients with MPA have gastrointestinal involvement, though the specific manifestations are not noted in published materials. Four percent of the patients with MPA experienced severe GI manifestations as defined by five-factor score criteria (92) to include GI bleeding, perforation, infarction, and pancreatitis. The presence of such severe GI manifestations was prognostic of an increased mortality rate as compared to patients with MPA without severe GI involvement (93). Ten percent of patients with GPA had at least one GI manifestation. In 5% of cases, the only symptom was abdominal pain; however, 0.3% (2 patients of 727) had GI perforation (90). In this cohort, the presence of GI symptoms did not influence the risk of death or disease relapse (90). Twenty percent of patients with EGPA had abdominal pain, and 6% had surgical abdomen. Only 2% were designated with severe vasculitis-related GI involvement (94).

TREATMENT

Treatment of GPA and MPA is largely similar, as major trials have enrolled patients with either disease. Treatment has primarily two phases: induction of remission followed by maintenance. For induction, the American College of Rheumatology and Vasculitis Foundation (ACR/VF) guidelines recommend rituximab over cyclophosphamide for patients with severe disease, for which GI involvement is a qualifying factor. For maintenance, the same guidelines recommend rituximab over methotrexate or azathioprine (95). Another expert group from the FVSG has general agreement but notes more equipoise between rituximab and cyclophosphamide for induction as well as rituximab as compared to other therapies for maintenance (96). Complement inhibition with medications like avacopan (C5a inhibitor) is an emerging adjunct treatment approach with the ability to potentially reduce the amount of glucocorticoids needed to control disease (97). If a medication is implicated as the cause of vasculitis, then that medication should be withdrawn and added to the "allergy list" of the patient to avoid future exposure.

As with MPA and GPA, treatment of EGPA proceeds in phases: induction and maintenance. The ACR/VF guidelines recommend induction with either rituximab or cyclophosphamide along with high-dose glucocorticoids for patients with severe (i.e., organ- or life-threatening) disease. Hence the presence of GI ischemia would disqualify the patient from receiving mepolizumab as initial therapy; this agent suppresses eosinophil production through targeting IL-5 and is favored for patients with a predominantly hypereosinophilic presentation when there is no concern for critical organ injury from vasculitis. For maintenance of remission, ACR/VF guidelines recommend methotrexate, azathioprine, or mycophenolate over mepolizumab or rituximab (95).

CAUSES OF SECONDARY GI VASCULITIS

Systemic Lupus Erythematosus

Systemic lupus erythematosus (SLE) can affect the GI tract and abdomen in several ways. Mesenteric vasculitis has been rarely reported in patients with SLE (98). Abdominal serositis, pancreatitis, and oral and/or perianal ulceration are other ways SLE can affect the GI tract, but it is less clear whether vasculitic injury is the primary mechanism in these cases.

Antiphospholipid syndrome (APLS), with or without SLE, is an important consideration in patients with multiple vascular beds affected or when thrombus is suspected or confirmed. Diagnosis is based on a persistently positive antiphospholipid antibody (lupus anticoagulant, anticardiolipin, or anti-beta-2-glycoprotein antibodies, generally greater than 40 units) in the setting of an arterial or venous thrombus or pregnancy morbidity. The risk of thrombosis is highest in those with a positive lupus anticoagulant as well as those who are double or triple positivity (99, 100). A particularly devastating form of APLS is known as catastrophic antiphospholipid syndrome and can affect multiple organ systems over a short amount of time.

Seronegative Spondyloarthropathy-Associated Vasculitis

While many forms of systemic vasculitis can develop gastrointestinal manifestations, primary forms of inflammatory bowel disease (IBD: Crohn's and ulcerative colitis) can also develop vasculitis. In a large, multicenter series, which included a literature review of prior published cases, the strongest association appears to be with large-vessel vasculitis, specifically TAK (101). Within this group, the diagnosis of IBD preceded the diagnosis of large-vessel vasculitis in 69% of cases, by a median of 4 years. Most of the patients with combined IBD and large-vessel vasculitis responded to TNF inhibitors. Compared to patients with isolated TAK, the group with TAK and IBD was more commonly Asian and diagnosed with TAK at a younger age (101). Other forms of vasculitis with concomitant IBD, reported in multiple cases, have included skin-limited vasculitis (both cutaneous PAN and leukocytoclastic vasculitis), ANCA associated vasculitis, IgA vasculitis, retinal vasculitis, and CNS vasculitis (101). Of note, medication-induced vasculitis should be considered in IBD patients presenting with cutaneous vasculitis, especially those on anti-TNF therapeutics (101).

Cryoglobulinemic Vasculitis

DEFINITION

A cryoglobulin is any immunoglobulin in plasma that remains soluble above 37°C and forms aggregates at lower temperatures. There are generally three types, two of which can cause vasculitis. Type 2 refers to a polyclonal collection of IgG molecules and another monoclonal immunoglobulin of another subtype. Type 3 refers to a polyclonal collection of immunoglobulins without enrichment of any large representation of any one clone. These two types can be referred to collectively as "mixed cryoglobulinemia." (By contrast, type 1 consists only of monoclonal immunoglobulin.) It can be difficult to test for cryoglobulins directly due to their temperature sensitivity, but in the correct clinical context, a patient with these specific lab values can be considered likely to have cryoglobulinemia: positive rheumatoid factor, normal C3, low C4.

EPIDEMIOLOGY

Historically, mixed cryoglobulinemia was mostly caused by HCV. But with new direct antiviral treatments, the prevalence of HCV has decreased, and non-HCV cryoglobulinemia is now more common than HCV-related cryoglobulinemia (102). Among patients with non-HCV cryoglobulinemia, autoimmune diseases are the most common causes, followed by hematologic disease and other infections. The most common autoimmune causes are systemic lupus erythematosus and Sjogren's disease. Across all etiologies of cryoglobulinemia, approximately 20% of patients with cryoglobulinemia develop cryoglobulinemic vasculitis (102).

GASTROINTESTINAL MANIFESTATIONS

In one study of 145 patients with noninfectious mixed cryoglobulinemic vasculitis, 87% had skin manifestations, most commonly palpable purpura, and approximately half had peripheral nerve involvement (55%) and joint involvement (42%). Gastrointestinal involvement was rare at

6%. However, GI involvement has been found to be a predictor of increased mortality, along with age greater than 65 years, pulmonary involvement, and renal failure (103, 104).

TREATMENT

In patients with virus-induced cryoglobulinemia, treatment of the causative infection is of primary importance. In patients without markers of severe or organ-threatening disease, no further treatment may be needed.

For patients with severe disease, marked by organ-threatening vasculitis, we strongly consider treatment with IV methylprednisolone followed by a 3-month course of oral prednisone along with rituximab. None of these immunosuppressive therapies should delay treatment of the underlying infection if there is one (105).

Drug-Induced Vasculitis

The primary ways in which ingested substances can cause vasculitis are hydralazine-associated ANCA-associated vasculitis (AAV) and levamisole-associated AAV, which are discussed in the section on AAV, and minocycline-associated PAN, which is discussed in the section on PAN.

Infection-Associated Vasculitis

The principle ways in which infection can cause vasculitis are HBV-associated PAN-like syndrome, which is discussed in the section on PAN, and through cryoglobulinemia, which is discussed in the section on cryoglobulinemic vasculitis.

NONINFLAMMATORY VASCULOPATHIES

Noninflammatory vasculopathy syndromes are often a challenge to distinguish from vasculitis in a clinical setting. No symptom or collection of symptoms is specific enough to distinguish the two categories, and imaging findings can be very similar in terms of "beading" and stenotic and aneurysmal disease. Even vascular "stranding" is not specific for vasculitis and can be seen with embolic phenomena. Typically, patients with a noninflammatory cause of ischemia will not have a history, exam findings, or laboratory results that indicate systemic inflammation. This is one reason

the high prevalence of weight loss and fever is so clinically helpful in the diagnosis of inflammatory vasculitides.

Atherosclerosis is perhaps the most common noninflammatory mimic of mesenteric vasculitis and should be high on a differential diagnosis in an older patient with typical cardiovascular disease risk factors such as tobacco use, diabetes, and hypertension. A high burden of calcific atherosclerosis on X-ray or computed tomographic imaging, particularly at the site of stenosis or aneurysm, would suggest atherosclerosis as an underlying cause for the ischemia (106).

Embolic or thrombotic phenomena are frequent mimics of abdominal vasculitis. The patient presenting with evidence of acute mesenteric ischemia should be evaluated for cardiac arrhythmia, most commonly atrial fibrillation. Thrombotic or thrombophilic disease like Factor V Leiden or Protein C or S deficiency can also be implicated (107). As described, if clot is discovered upon evaluation, then two important inflammatory etiologies to consider are Behçet disease (ultimately a clinical diagnosis in the setting of the typical oral and genital lesions and other supportive findings) and the antiphospholipid syndrome (which can be confirmed with serologic testing).

Vasoconstrictive medications must be considered in a patient with stenotic vascular disease on imaging felt to be causing ischemic symptoms. A careful history would reveal exposure to a substance like cocaine or ergots that are known to constrict vessels. Confirmatory blood or urine analysis can be done if considered in a timely manner. Case reports have attributed Raynaud phenomenon (RP) to stimulant medications prescribed for attention-deficit hyperactivity disorder (108). Additionally, one small, retrospective case-control analysis found that stimulant medication use was more common among children with RP than among those without (109).

Noninflammatory vasculopathies affecting connective tissue are a particular challenge to the clinician, as they can affect multiple vascular beds in the manner of a systemic process. Patients with polygenic diseases such as fibromuscular dysplasia (FMD) and segmental arterial mediolysis (SAM) typically have focal arterial lesions that are radiographically similar to vasculitic lesions, although there are subtle differences that an experienced radiologist may identify. Monogenic syndromes

Table 8.1 GI Manifestations of Vasculitis Syndromes

	Mouth	Esophagus	Stomach	Small intestine	Large intestine	Spleen	Pancreas	Hepatobiliary
LVV								
TAK	–	–	–	common (77)	common (65, 77)	Uncommon (77)	Uncommon (77)	rare—PSC (110)
GCA	rare—tongue necrosis (67)	–	–	common (66)	Common (66)	–	–	–
MVV								
PAN	–	–	Rare perforation (27)	Rare perforation (27)	Rare perforation (27)	–	Rare pancreatitis (27)	–
SVV								
MPA	–	–	Uncommon abdominal pain, rare perforation (93)	–	–	–	–	–
GPA	–	–	Uncommon abdominal pain, rare perforation (90)	–	–	–	–	–
eGPA			Common abdominal pain, rare perforation (94)		Ulceration			
IgA					Typical abdominal pain, common bleeding and diarrhea, uncommon perforation or ileus (13)		Rare pancreatitis (13)	
Cryoglobulinemic			Uncommon abdominal pain	Uncommon abdominal pain (104)				
VVV								
Behçet	Typical ulcers (46)		Common abdominal pain (46)	Uncommon duodenal, jejunal, or ileal ulcers (46)	Common ileocecal ulcers (46)			Rare BCS (46)
Systemic autoimmune diseases that can cause secondary vasculitis								
SLE	–	–	–	Rare SMA involvement (98)	–	–	–	–
RA	–	–	–	Rare abdominal pain, ischemic ulcers, perforation, infarction (111)	–	–	–	–

Table 8.1 Generally, large-vessel vasculitis (LVV) and medium-vessel vasculitis (MVV) affect the GI tract when they cause obstruction or destruction of a vessel that supplies a gut segment with blood, causing ischemia, possible necrosis, and perforation. Generally, small-vessel vasculitis (SVV) causes microscopic obstruction of small blood vessels leading to ulceration which can also progress to necrosis and perforation. "typical": more than half of patients with the vasculitis syndrome have the noted part of the GI tract affected; "common": 10% to 50%; "uncommon": 1% to 10%; "rare": < 1%; PSC: primary sclerosing cholangitis; BCS: Budd–Chiari Syndrome, SMA: superior mesenteric artery

like vascular Ehlers-Danlos syndrome (vEDS), Marfan syndrome, and Loeys-Dietz syndrome are less-common but important mimics to consider if the patient has predominantly aneurysmal disease. A careful physical examination might reveal non-vascular stigmata suggestive of these syndromes, such as the typical facial features of Loeys-Dietz syndrome, the habitus of a patient with Marfan syndrome, or the thin, almost translucent skin of a patient with vEDS. Commercially available genetic testing panels to confirm these diagnoses are rapidly progressing in sensitivity and affordability. As discussed, a history that reveals constitutional symptoms should prompt the clinician to evaluate further for autoimmune disease as the etiology.

CONCLUSION

Vasculitis encompasses a myriad of primary and secondary disease processes, as well as rare drug effects, many of which have been reported to cause manifestations in the GI tract. Table 8.1 summarizes the various GI findings of the major subtypes of vasculitis managed in rheumatology. Many of these can have serious sequalae, and a high index of suspicion is required by the managing teams for early diagnosis and intervention to improve outcomes.

REFERENCES

1. Jennette JC, Falk RJ, Bacon PA et al. 2012 revised international chapel hill consensus conference nomenclature of vasculitides. *Arthritis Rheum.* 2013;65(1):1–11.
2. Matteson EL. History of vasculitis: The life and work of Adolf Kussmaul. *Cleve Clin J Med.* 2012;79(Suppl 3):S54–6.
3. Kussmaul A. Uber eine nicht bisher beschriebene eigenthumliche Arterienerkrankung (Periarteritis nodosa), die mit Morbus Brightii und rapid fortschreitender allgemeiner Muskelahmung einhergeht. *Dtsch Arch Klin Med.* 1866;1:484–518.
4. Ozen S, Pistorio A, Iusan SM et al. EULAR/PRINTO/PRES criteria for Henoch-Schonlein purpura, childhood polyarteritis nodosa, childhood Wegener granulomatosis and childhood Takayasu arteritis: Ankara 2008: Part II: Final classification criteria. *Ann Rheum Dis.* 2010;69(5):798–806.
5. Mills JA, Michel BA, Bloch DA et al. The American college of rheumatology 1990 criteria for the classification of Henoch-Schönlein purpura. *Arthritis Rheum.* 2010;33(8):1114–21.
6. Aalberse J, Dolman K, Ramnath G et al. Henoch Schonlein purpura in children: An epidemiological study among Dutch paediatricians on incidence and diagnostic criteria. *Ann Rheum Dis.* 2007;66(12):1648–50.
7. Piram M, Maldini C, Biscardi S et al. Incidence of IgA vasculitis in children estimated by four-source capture—Recapture analysis: A population-based study. *Rheumatol.* 2017;56(8):1358–66.
8. Calviño MC, Llorca J, García-Porrúa C et al. Henoch-Schönlein purpura in children from Northwestern Spain: A 20-year epidemiologic and clinical study. *Med* (Baltimore). 2001;80(5):279–90.
9. Yang YH, Hung CF, Hsu CR et al. A nationwide survey on epidemiological characteristics of childhood Henoch—Schönlein purpura in Taiwan. *Rheumatol.* 2005;44(5):618–22.
10. Gardner-Medwin JM, Dolezalova P, Cummins C et al. Incidence of Henoch-Schonlein purpura, Kawasaki disease, and rare vasculitides in children of different ethnic origins. *Lancet.* 2002;360(9341):1197–202.
11. Piram M, Mahr A. Epidemiology of immunoglobulin a vasculitis (Henoch—Schönlein): Current state of knowledge. *Curr Opin Rheumatol.* 2013;25(2):171–8.
12. Hočevar A, Rotar Z, Ostrovršnik J et al. Incidence of IgA vasculitis in the adult Slovenian population. *Br J Dermatol.* 2014;171(3):524–7.
13. Audemard-Verger A, Pillebout E, Amoura Z et al. Gastrointestinal involvement in adult IgA vasculitis (Henoch-Schönlein purpura): Updated picture from a French multicentre and retrospective series of 260 cases. *Rheumatol.* 2020;59(10):3050–7.
14. Audemard-Verger A, Terrier B, Dechartres A et al. Characteristics and management of IgA vasculitis (Henoch-Schönlein) in adults: Data from 260 patients included in a French multicenter retrospective survey:

IgA vasculitis in adults. *Arthritis Rheumatol.* 2017;69(9):1862–70.

15. Pillebout E, Alberti C, Guillevin L et al. Addition of cyclophosphamide to steroids provides no benefit compared with steroids alone in treating adult patients with severe Henoch Schönlein purpura. *Kidney Int.* 2010;78(5):495–502.

16. Maritati F, Fenoglio R, Pillebout E et al. Brief report: Rituximab for the treatment of adult-onset IgA vasculitis (Henoch-Schönlein). *Arthritis Rheumatol.* 2018;70(1):109–14.

17. Oni L, Sampath S. Childhood IgA vasculitis (Henoch Schonlein purpura)—Advances and knowledge gaps. *Front Pediatr.* 2019;7:257.

18. Ozen S, Marks SD, Brogan P et al. European consensus-based recommendations for diagnosis and treatment of immunoglobulin a vasculitis—The share initiative. *Rheumatol.* 2019;58(9):1607–16.

19. Pillebout E, Sunderkötter C. IgA vasculitis. *Semin Immunopathol.* 2021;43(5):729–38.

20. Jennette JC, Falk RJ, Andrassy K et al. Nomenclature of systemic vasculitides. *Arthritis Rheum.* 1994;37(2):187–92.

21. Trepo C, Thivolet J. Hepatitis associated antigen and Periarteritis Nodosa (PAN). *Vox Sang.* 1970;19(3):410–11.

22. Lightfoot RW, Michel BA, Bloch DA et al. The American college of rheumatology 1990 criteria for the classification of polyarteritis nodosa. *Arthritis Rheum.* 1990;33(8):1088–93.

23. Kanecki K, Nitsch-Osuch A, Gorynski P et al. Polyarteritis nodosa: Decreasing incidence in Poland. *Arch Med Sci.* 2019;15(5):1308–12. https://doi.org/10.5114/aoms.2017.68407

24. Watts RA. Geoepidemiology of systemic vasculitis: Comparison of the incidence in two regions of Europe. *Ann Rheum Dis.* 2001;60(2):170–2.

25. Watts RA, Lane SE, Bentham G et al. Epidemiology of systemic vasculitis: A ten-year study in the United Kingdom. *Arthritis Rheum.* 2000;43(2):414.

26. Alibaz-Oner F, Koster MJ, Crowson CS et al. Clinical spectrum of medium-sized vessel vasculitis. *Arthritis Care Res.* 2017;69(6):884–91.

27. Pagnoux C, Seror R, Henegar C et al. Clinical features and outcomes in 348 patients with polyarteritis nodosa: A systematic retrospective study of patients diagnosed between 1963 and 2005 and entered into the French vasculitis study group database. *Arthritis Rheum.* 2010;62(2):616–26.

28. Chung SA, Gorelik M, Langford CA et al. 2021 American college of rheumatology/vasculitis foundation guideline for the management of polyarteritis nodosa. *Arthritis Care Res.* 2021;73(8):1061–70.

29. Saadoun D, Terrier B, Semoun O et al. Hepatitis C virus-associated polyarteritis nodosa. *Arthritis Care Res.* 2011;63(3):427–35.

30. Patel N, Patel N, Khan T et al. HIV infection and clinical spectrum of associated vasculitides. *Curr Rheumatol Rep.* 2011;13(6):506–12.

31. Kermani TA, Ham EK, Camilleri MJ et al. Polyarteritis nodosa-like vasculitis in association with minocycline use: A single-center case series. *Semin Arthritis Rheum.* 2012;42(2):213–21.

32. Guillevin L, Mahr A, Cohen P et al. Short-term corticosteroids then lamivudine and plasma exchanges to treat hepatitis B virus-related polyarteritis nodosa. *Arthritis Rheum.* 2004;51(3):482–7.

33. Ancient missense mutations in a new member of the RoRet gene family are likely to cause familial Mediterranean fever: The international FMF consortium. *Cell.* 1997;90(4):797–807.

34. Familial Mediterranean Fever (FMF) in Turkey: Results of a nationwide multicenter study. *Med (Baltimore).* 2005;84(1):1–11.

35. Daniels M, Shohat T, Brenner-Ullman A et al. Familial Mediterranean fever: High gene frequency among the non-Ashkenazic and Ashkenazic Jewish populations in Israel. *Am J Med Genet.* 1995;55(3):311–14.

36. Sarkisian T, Ajrapetian H, Beglarian A et al. Familial Mediterranean fever in Armenian population. *Georgian Med News.* 2008;(156):105–11.

37. Ben-Chetrit E, Touitou I. Familial Mediterranean fever in the world. *Arthritis Rheum.* 2009;61(10):1447–53.

38. Ben-Chetrit E, Yazici H. Familial Mediterranean fever: Different faces around the world. *Clin Exp Rheumatol.* 2019;37 Suppl 121(6):18–22.

39. Babaoglu H, Varan O, Kucuk H et al. Effectiveness of canakinumab in colchicine- and anakinra-resistant or-intolerant adult familial Mediterranean fever patients: A single-center real-life study. *JCR J Clin Rheumatol.* 2020;26(1):7–13.

40. Ozdogan H, Arisoy N, Kasapçapur O et al. Vasculitis in familial Mediterranean fever. *J Rheumatol.* 1997;24(2):323–7.

41. Abbara S, Monfort JB, Savey L et al. Vasculitis and familial Mediterranean fever: Description of 22 French adults from the juvenile inflammatory rheumatism cohort. *Front Med.* 2022;9:1000167.

42. Zhou Q, Yang D, Ombrello AK et al. Early-onset stroke and vasculopathy associated with mutations in ADA2. *N Engl J Med.* 2014;370(10):911–20.

43. Navon Elkan P, Pierce SB, Segel R et al. Mutant adenosine deaminase 2 in a polyarteritis nodosa vasculopathy. *N Engl J Med.* 2014;370(10):921–31.

44. Wang XF, Calame K. SV40 enhancer-binding factors are required at the establishment but not the maintenance step of enhancer-dependent transcriptional activation. *Cell.* 1986;47(2):241–7.

45. Deuitch NT, Yang D, Lee PY et al. TNF inhibition in vasculitis management in adenosine deaminase 2 deficiency (DADA2). *J Allergy Clin Immunol.* 2022;149(5):1812–16. e6.

46. Yazici Y, Hatemi G, Bodaghi B et al. Behçet syndrome. *Nat Rev Dis Primer.* 2021;7(1):1–14.

47. Mohammad A, Mandl T, Sturfelt G et al. Incidence, prevalence and clinical characteristics of Behçet's disease in southern Sweden. *Rheumatol.* 2013;52(2):304–10.

48. Calamia KT, Wilson FC, Icen M et al. Epidemiology and clinical characteristics of Behçet's disease in the US: A population-based study. *Arthritis Rheum.* 2009;61(5):600–4.

49. Ohno S, Aoki K, Sugiura S et al. Letter: HL-A5 and Behçet's disease. *Lancet Lond Engl.* 1973;2(7842):1383–4.

50. Criteria for diagnosis of Behçet's disease: International study group for Behçet's disease. *Lancet Lond Engl.* 1990;335(8697):1078–80.

51. Bettiol A, Prisco D, Emmi G. Behçet: The syndrome. *Rheumatol.* 2020;59(Suppl 3):iii101–7.

52. International Team for the Revision of the International Criteria for Behçet's Disease (ITR-ICBD), Davatchi F, Assaad-Khalil S et al. The International Criteria for Behçet's Disease (ICBD): A collaborative study of 27 countries on the sensitivity and specificity of the new criteria. *J Eur Acad Dermatol Venereol.* 2014;28(3):338–47.

53. Kural-Seyahi E, Fresko I, Seyahi N et al. The long-term mortality and morbidity of Behçet syndrome: A 2-decade outcome survey of 387 patients followed at a dedicated center. *Med* (Baltimore). 2003;82(1):60–76.

54. Lee JH, Cheon JH, Jeon SW et al. Efficacy of infliximab in intestinal Behçet's disease: A Korean multicenter retrospective study. *Inflamm Bowel Dis.* Published online 2013 May:1.

55. Cheon JH, Kim WH. An update on the diagnosis, treatment, and prognosis of intestinal Behçet's disease. *Curr Opin Rheumatol.* 2015;27(1):24–31.

56. Hatemi I, Hatemi G, Çelik AF. Gastrointestinal involvement in Behçet disease. *Rheum Dis Clin N Am.* 2018;44(1):45–64.

57. Tascilar K, Melikoglu M, Ugurlu S et al. Vascular involvement in Behçet's syndrome: A retrospective analysis of associations and the time course. *Rheumatol.* 2014;53(11):2018–22.

58. Hatemi G, Christensen R, Bang D et al. 2018 update of the EULAR recommendations for the management of Behçet's syndrome. *Ann Rheum Dis.* Published online 2018 Apr 6. https://doi.org/10.1136/annrheumdis-2018-213225

59. Hatemi G, Mahr A, Ishigatsubo Y et al. Trial of apremilast for oral ulcers in Behçet's syndrome. *N Engl J Med.* 2019;381(20):1918–28.

60. Hatemi G, Melikoglu M, Tunc R et al. Apremilast for Behçet's syndrome—A

phase 2, placebo-controlled study. *N Engl J Med.* 2015;372(16):1510–18.

61. Melikoglu M, Fresko I, Mat C et al. Short-term trial of etanercept in Behçet's disease: A double blind, placebo controlled study. *J Rheumatol.* 2005;32(1):98–105.

62. Li KJ, Semenov D, Turk M et al. A meta-analysis of the epidemiology of giant cell arteritis across time and space. *Arthritis Res Ther.* 2021;23(1):82.

63. Gruener AM, Poostchi A, Carey AR et al. Association of giant cell arteritis with race. *JAMA Ophthalmol.* 2019;137(10):1175–9.

64. Blockmans D, de Ceuninck L, Vanderschueren S et al. Repetitive 18F-fluorodeoxyglucose positron emission tomography in giant cell arteritis: A prospective study of 35 patients. *Arthritis Rheum.* 2006;55(1):131–7.

65. Gribbons KB, Ponte C, Carette S et al. Patterns of arterial disease in Takayasu arteritis and giant cell arteritis. *Arthritis Care Res.* 2020;72(11):1615–24.

66. Grayson PC, Maksimowicz-McKinnon K, Clark TM et al. Distribution of arterial lesions in Takayasu's arteritis and giant cell arteritis. *Ann Rheum Dis.* 2012;71(8):1329–34.

67. Brodmann M, Dorr A, Hafner F et al. Tongue necrosis as first symptom of Giant Cell Arteritis (GCA). *Clin Rheumatol.* 2009;28(S1):47–9.

68. Henderson AH. Tongue pain with giant cell arteritis. *BMJ.* 1967;4(5575):337.

69. Maz M, Chung SA, Abril A et al. 2021 American college of rheumatology/vasculitis foundation guideline for the management of giant cell arteritis and Takayasu arteritis. *Arthritis Care Res.* 2021;73(8):1071–87.

70. Curtis JR, Perez-Gutthann S, Suissa S et al. Tocilizumab in rheumatoid arthritis: A case study of safety evaluations of a large postmarketing data set from multiple data sources. *Semin Arthritis Rheum.* 2015;44(4):381–8.

71. Rempenault C, Lukas C, Combe B et al. Risk of diverticulitis and gastrointestinal perforation in rheumatoid arthritis treated with tocilizumab compared to rituximab or abatacept. *Rheumatol.* 2022;61(3):953–62.

72. Stone JH, Han J, Aringer M et al. Long-term effect of tocilizumab in patients with giant cell arteritis: Open-label extension phase of the Giant Cell Arteritis Actemra (GiACTA) trial. *Lancet Rheumatol.* 2021;3(5):e328–36.

73. Rutter M, Bowley J, Lanyon PC et al. A systematic review and meta-analysis of the incidence rate of Takayasu arteritis. *Rheumatol.* 2021;60(11):4982–90.

74. Park SJ, Kim HJ, Park H et al. Incidence, prevalence, mortality and causes of death in Takayasu arteritis in Korea—A nationwide, population-based study. *Int J Cardiol.* 2017;235:100–4.

75. Dammacco F, Cirulli A, Simeone A et al. Takayasu arteritis: A cohort of Italian patients and recent pathogenetic and therapeutic advances. *Clin Exp Med.* 2021;21(1):49–62.

76. Schmidt J, Kermani TA, Bacani AK et al. Diagnostic features, treatment, and outcomes of Takayasu arteritis in a US cohort of 126 patients. *Mayo Clin Proc.* 2013;88(8):822–30.

77. Sanchez-Alvarez C, Mertz LE, Thomas CS et al. Demographic, clinical, and radiologic characteristics of a cohort of patients with Takayasu arteritis. *Am J Med.* 2019;132(5):647–51.

78. Jiang Z, Lefebvre F, Ross C et al. Variations in Takayasu arteritis characteristics in a cohort of patients with different racial backgrounds. *Semin Arthritis Rheum.* 2022;53:151971.

79. Comarmond C, Biard L, Lambert M et al. Long-term outcomes and prognostic factors of complications in Takayasu arteritis: A multicenter study of 318 patients. *Circulation.* 2017;136(12):1114–22.

80. Hoffman GS, Leavitt RY, Kerr GS et al. Treatment of glucocorticoid-resistant or relapsing Takayasu arteritis with methotrexate. *Arthritis Rheum.* 1994;37(4):578–82.

81. Hoffman GS, Merkel PA, Brasington RD et al. Anti-tumor necrosis factor therapy in patients with difficult to treat Takayasu arteritis. *Arthritis Rheum.* 2004;50(7):2296–304.

82. Nakaoka Y, Isobe M, Takei S et al. Efficacy and safety of tocilizumab in patients with refractory Takayasu arteritis: Results from a randomised, double-blind,

placebo-controlled, phase 3 trial in Japan (the TAKT study). *Ann Rheum Dis.* 2018;77(3):348–54.

83. Langford CA, Cuthbertson D, Ytterberg SR et al. A randomized, double-blind trial of abatacept (CTLA-4Ig) for the treatment of giant cell arteritis. *Arthritis Rheumatol.* 2017;69(4):837–45.

84. Kong X, Sun Y, Dai X et al. Treatment efficacy and safety of tofacitinib versus methotrexate in Takayasu arteritis: A prospective observational study. *Ann Rheum Dis.* 2022;81(1):117–23.

85. Mahr A, Katsahian S, Varet H et al. Revisiting the classification of clinical phenotypes of anti-neutrophil cytoplasmic antibody-associated vasculitis: A cluster analysis. *Ann Rheum Dis.* 2013;72(6):1003–10.

86. Gross RL, Brucker J, Bahce-Altuntas A et al. A novel cutaneous vasculitis syndrome induced by levamisole-contaminated cocaine. *Clin Rheumatol.* 2011;30(10):1385–92.

87. Choi HK, Merkel PA, Walker AM et al. Drug-associated antineutrophil cytoplasmic antibody-positive vasculitis: Prevalence among patients with high titers of antimyeloperoxidase antibodies. *Arthritis Rheum.* 2000;43(2):405–13.

88. Schirmer JH, Wright MN, Vonthein R et al. Clinical presentation and long-term outcome of 144 patients with microscopic polyangiitis in a monocentric German cohort. *Rheumatol Oxf Engl.* 2016;55(1):71–9.

89. Hoffman GS, Kerr GS, Leavitt RY et al. Wegener granulomatosis: An analysis of 158 patients. *Ann Intern Med.* 1992;116(6):488–98.

90. Puéchal X, Iudici M, Pagnoux C et al. Comparative study of granulomatosis with polyangiitis subsets according to ANCA status: Data from the French vasculitis study group registry. *RMD Open.* 2022;8(1):e002160.

91. Mohammad AJ. An update on the epidemiology of ANCA-associated vasculitis. *Rheumatol.* 2020;59(Suppl 3):iii42–50.

92. Guillevin L, Lhote F, Gayraud M et al. Prognostic factors in polyarteritis nodosa and Churg-Strauss syndrome a prospective study in 342 patients. *Med* (Baltimore). 1996;75(1):17–28.

93. Nguyen Y, Pagnoux C, Karras A et al. Microscopic polyangiitis: Clinical characteristics and long-term outcomes of 378 patients from the French vasculitis study group registry. *J Autoimmun.* 2020;112:102467.

94. Comarmond C, Pagnoux C, Khellaf M et al. Eosinophilic granulomatosis with polyangiitis (Churg-Strauss): Clinical characteristics and long-term follow-up of the 383 patients enrolled in the French vasculitis study group cohort. *Arthritis Rheum.* 2013;65(1):270–81.

95. Chung SA, Langford CA, Maz M et al. 2021 American college of rheumatology/vasculitis foundation guideline for the management of antineutrophil cytoplasmic antibody—Associated vasculitis. *Arthritis Rheumatol.* 2021;73(8):1366–83.

96. Terrier B, Charles P, Aumaître O et al. ANCA-associated vasculitides: Recommendations of the French vasculitis study group on the use of immunosuppressants and biotherapies for remission induction and maintenance. *Presse Médicale.* 2020;49(3):104031.

97. Jayne DRW, Merkel PA, Schall TJ et al. Avacopan for the treatment of ANCA-associated vasculitis. *N Engl J Med.* 2021;384(7):599–609.

98. Fotis L, Baszis KW, French AR et al. Mesenteric vasculitis in children with systemic lupus erythematosus. *Clin Rheumatol.* 2016;35(3):785–93.

99. Wahl DG, Guillemin F, de Maistre E et al. Risk for venous thrombosis related to antiphospholipid antibodies in systemic lupus erythematosus—A meta-analysis. *Lupus.* 1997;6(5):467–73.

100. Mustonen P, Lehtonen KV, Javela K et al. Persistent antiphospholipid antibody (aPL) in asymptomatic carriers as a risk factor for future thrombotic events: A nationwide prospective study. *Lupus.* 2014;23(14):1468–76.

101. Sy A, Khalidi N, Dehghan N et al. Vasculitis in patients with inflammatory bowel diseases: A study of 32 patients and systematic review of the literature. *Semin Arthritis Rheum.* 2016;45(4):475–82.

102. Silva F, Pinto C, Barbosa A et al. New insights in cryoglobulinemic vasculitis. *J Autoimmun.* 2019;105:102313.

103. Terrier B, Carrat F, Krastinova E et al. Prognostic factors of survival in patients with non-infectious mixed cryoglobulinaemia vasculitis: Data from 242 cases included in the CryoVas survey. *Ann Rheum Dis.* 2013;72(3):374–80.

104. Terrier B, Marie I, Launay D et al. Predictors of early relapse in patients with non-infectious mixed cryoglobulinemia vasculitis: Results from the French nationwide CryoVas survey. *Autoimmun Rev.* 2014;13(6):630–4.

105. Comarmond C, Cacoub P, Saadoun D. Treatment of chronic hepatitis C-associated cryoglobulinemia vasculitis at the era of direct-acting antivirals. *Ther Adv Gastroenterol.* 2020;13:175628482094261.

106. Nienhuis PH, van Praagh GD, Glaudemans AWJM et al. A review on the value of imaging in differentiating between large vessel vasculitis and atherosclerosis. *J Pers Med.* 2021;11(3):236.

107. Lim MY, Moll S. Thrombophilia. *Vasc Med.* 2015;20(2):193–6.

108. Gupta M. Rare side effects of stimulants: Raynaud's phenomenon. *Prim Care Companion CNS Disord.* 2021;23(5).

109. Goldman W, Seltzer R, Reuman P. Association between treatment with central nervous system stimulants and Raynaud's syndrome in children: A retrospective case—Control study of rheumatology patients. *Arthritis Rheum.* 2008;58(2):563–6.

110. Mulinacci G, Palermo A, Cristoferi L et al. Takayasu arteritis and primary sclerosing cholangitis: A casual association or different phenotypes of the same disease? *J Transl Autoimmun.* 2021;4:100124.

111. Craig E, Cappelli LC. Gastrointestinal and hepatic disease in rheumatoid arthritis. *Rheum Dis Clin N Am.* 2018;44(1):89–111.

9

Nutrition and Diet for Patients with Rheumatic Disease

CHELSEA THOMPSON AND DEJAN MICIC

INTRODUCTION

Over 4 years of medical school, less than 20 hours of time is dedicated to nutritional education (1). Residency and fellowship training programs typically offer no mandatory or supplemental instruction concerning the impact of nutrition on disease activity.

However, many patients are curious about how dietary factors influence their disease. In this chapter, we will review the vast body of literature examining the impact of diet in various rheumatic diseases and discuss the risks and consequences of malnutrition in rheumatic diseases with concurrent gastrointestinal comorbidities.

RHEUMATOID ARTHRITIS

The worldwide incidence of rheumatoid arthritis (RA) is rising (2). This increase in RA incidence has been associated with the increased and widespread adoption of Western dietary practices, which include regular consumption of ultraprocessed foods and sugary beverages and low intake of dietary fiber (3).

Specific aspects of western dietary patterns in excess have emerged as risk factors for developing RA. In prospective studies, daily sodium intake of greater than 4 grams, daily processed meat intake, and the consumption of one or more sugar-sweetened beverage per day have been associated with an increased likelihood for RA (4–6). Diet sodas appear to have no correlational relationship to development of RA (5).

Dietary Patterns and Disease Activity in Rheumatoid Arthritis: Vegan Diet

Prior to the availability of biologic disease-modifying antirheumatic drugs (bDMARD) for the treatment of RA, European rheumatologists and health advocates frequently recommended a vegan diet to ameliorate symptoms of RA (7). Multiple randomized controlled trials (RCTs) exploring the impact of vegan and vegetarian-style diets on RA disease activity were published during this era, between 1979 and 2001. The pooled results of four Scandinavian RCTs (excluding one RCT with a "raw" vegan diet intervention) demonstrate a modest subjective improvement in joint pain for patients with RA on a vegan or vegetarian diet (8–11). Two of these trials demonstrated a statistically significant decrease in objective measures of disease activity with the vegan diet intervention (8, 9). Only one study of the group used the disease activity measure "ACR 20," which has become the standard measure for efficacy in pharmaceutical trials for RA treatment, as a primary outcome measure (8).

The only randomized controlled trial to explore a raw vegan diet, which relies on sprouted grains and fermented foods for key nutrients, did not show objective improvements in RA disease activity compared to the control group. Over one-third

DOI: 10.1201/9781003367307-9

of patients in the raw vegan group had to stop the intervention early due to gastrointestinal upset (12).

Ultimately, the conclusion that vegan diets could eliminate the symptoms of RA and reverse disease activity proved overstated. There are no RCTs exploring the impact of dietary patterns on RA disease activity between 2004 and 2019, likely due to the successful development of various bDMARDS for the treatment of RA.

However, a renewed interest in diet for the adjunctive treatment of RA is demonstrated by the publication of multiple dietary intervention studies for RA after 2020 Table 9.1.

Neil Barnard, who is not a rheumatologist, published a randomized crossover study comparing a vegan dietary intervention to a placebo "supplement" intervention in 44 women with rheumatoid arthritis from the Washington, D.C., area. The participants were randomized to first follow either a vegan diet or to take a daily placebo supplement for 4 months and then switch study arms following the completion of a multiweek "washout" period. At the conclusion of the vegan diet, participants had a statistically significant improvement in DAS28-ESR scores by an average of 1.9 points, from 4.5 to 2.6 (13). This is notably the only RA dietary intervention study to include African American participants.

Dietary Patterns and Disease Activity in Rheumatoid Arthritis: Mediterranean Diet

The Mediterranean diet (MD) has shown benefit for primary and secondary cardiovascular disease prevention (14, 15). This dietary pattern eliminates processed foods, emphasizes multiple servings of fruits, vegetables, and whole grains, and encourages the consumption of oily fish two to five times per week (16). Polyunsaturated fat consumption through the addition of up to 4 tablespoons of olive oil per day is also an important component of this dietary pattern (15).

The first RCT exploring the impact of a Mediterranean-style diet for RA was published in 2003. The participants, recruited from a Swedish rheumatology clinic, received up to two meals daily during the 3-month study period as well as instructions for how to prepare meals in the MD style on their own time. Those randomized to the MD group demonstrated improvement in DAS28 scores compared to the control group following a standard Swedish diet (17).

A more recent rigorously designed, double blind, randomized control crossover study published in 2020 demonstrated modest improvement in disease activity scores for RA after an MD intervention period compared to the period after a control diet intervention (18). During the intervention period, participants received "fiber" packets containing the key ingredients to construct meals and snacks according to the MD. These ingredients included fish, whole-grain bread, and low-fat yogurt. During the control arm of the study, participants received isocaloric "protein" packets that were meant to mimic the contents of a standard Swedish diet that included fruit juice, butter, chicken, red meat, and white bread. Researchers noted that "responders" to the dietary intervention had higher baseline disease activity scores (DAS28-ESR) by an average of 1.5 points compared to the MD intervention "nonresponders."

The possible synergistic effects of a MD plus rigorous exercise for RA disease activity was demonstrated in a recent RCT from Mexico City, in which 144 female participants with well-controlled RA (mean DAS28-ESR score of 3.2) were randomized into one of four groups: MD plus intensive exercise, intensive exercise alone, MD alone, or no intervention. Those in the MD group met with a nutritionist and were provided with sample recipes to cook on their own time. Exercise took place twice a week for 90-minute sessions at a local gym, consisting of stretching, aerobic activity, strength training, and a group sport activity. Quality-of-life measures were highest in the MD plus exercise group at the end of the 3-month intervention period. MD alone increased quality of life compared to the control group with no interventions, but exercise alone had a more pronounced effect on quality of life than MD alone (19).

Dietary Patterns and Disease Activity in Rheumatoid Arthritis: Ketogenic Diet

Trials examining the impact of a ketogenic dietary pattern for rheumatoid arthritis fail to demonstrate either subjective or objective improvement in disease activity (20, 21).

Table 9.1 Dietary Randomized Controlled Trials for RA

Country	Publication Year	Authors	Intervention Group	Significant outcomes	Conclusions
Sweden	1979	Sköldstam L, Larsson L, Lindström FD	16 RA patients fast for 7–10 days, followed by vegetarian diet for 9 weeks	Subjective pain was reported in 5/15 during the fast but only 1/15 after 9 weeks on vegetarian diet	Fasting can induce short-term subjective changes
Sweden	1986	Sköldstam, L	20 RA patients fast for 7–10 days, followed by vegan diet for 4–5 months	No significant changes were observed between groups after 1 month.	No short-term changes were observed
Norway	1991	Kjeldsen-Kragh J, Haugen M, Borchgrevink CF, et al.	27 RA patients fast for 7–10 days followed by 3.5 months of a vegan diet and vegetarian for the rest of the year	Intervention group had improvements in subjective pain scores as well as reduced CRP and ESR at 4 weeks up until the end of the intervention	Fasting, followed by sustained, long-term dietary intervention shows benefit at 1 year
Finland	1998	Nenonen, M, et al.	19 patients with RA completed at least 2 months of a planned 3-month intervention of raw vegan diet, including a daily sprouted wheat drink	No statistically significant improvement in DAS28 between control and intervention groups at the end of the study. At least 8 patients stopped the study prior to 3 months due to GI upsent	A raw vegan diet may cause GI upset and should not be recommended for every patient
Sweden	2001	Hafstrom, et al.	22 patients followed gluten-free vegan diet for 1 year and 25 patients folllowed a control diet	At 6 months, 50% and at 12 months 40% met ACR20 criteria for improvement in the intervention group compared to 8% and 4% at 6 and 12 months, respectively. Responders to the diet had decreased gliadin antibodies during the experiment	Overall vegan diet was superior to control. Responders to the dietary intervention had decreasing gliadin antibody levels throughout the trial, suggesting food sensitivities that are not clinically apparent may mediate diet response.

(Continued)

Table 9.1 (Continued) Dietary Randomized Controlled Trials for RA

Country	Publication Year	Authors	Intervention Group	Significant outcomes	Conclusions
Sweden	2003	Sköldstam et al.	Mediterranean diet vs. control diet for 3 months. Patients were fed two meals daily during the week at the clinic canteen	Statistically significant decrease in DAS28 in the Mediterranean group compared to the control group at the end of the study	Mediterranean diet can have beneficial effects on RA disease activity as measured by DAS28
Sweden (ADIRA)	2020	Vadell et al.	50 RA patients were randomized to a Mediterranean Diet vs. control diet for 10 weeks with a 3-month washout period between diets	DAS28 significantly improved after the diet period as compared to the control period	Responders to the diet had an average DAS28 score of 4.5, whereas nonresponders had an average DAS28 of 3.0
Mexico City	2020	Garcia-Morales, et al.	130 patients were randomized to a MD-plus-exercise program, exercise alone, MD alone, or a control group	Globally, MD and exercise improved SF36 scores significantly after 6 months but at the same level as intensive exercise alone. MD alone improved SF36 scores after 6 months significantly but not to the effect of exercise alone or diet plus exercise.	MD alone did not improve measures of health in a manner that was statistically significant, but the combination of diet and exercise had the most significant impacts.
Germany (NutriFast)	2022	Hartman, et al.	50 patients were randomized to a 7-day fast followed by a vegan diet for 3 months or a Mediterranean-style anti-inflammatory diet	Significant improvement at the end of the 3 months in terms of DAS28, but no one group was superior to the other, except at the 1-week mark, when DAS28 was superior in the fasting group	Fasting can quickly improve disease activity in RA. Both MD and vegan dietary patterns significantly improve disease activity in RA patients.

Washington, D.C.	2022	Barnard, N. et al.	44 female RA patients in Washington, D.C., were randomized to placebo supplement or vegan diet for 4 months and then switched treatment arms after a 4-week washout period	Significant decrease in DAS after the treatment arm by 1.9, and 1.5 when adjusted for medication changes	Vegan diet led to significant improvement in disease activity. Mean DAS28 at the start of the vegan diet was 4.5, higher than other trials. Compared to ADIRA, higher average DAS28 activity scores, and increased overall response to intervention.

Dietary Patterns and Disease Activity in Rheumatoid Arthritis: Conclusions

At this time, the American College of Rheumatology (ACR) has conditionally recommended that all patient's with RA follow a "Mediterranean-style" dietary pattern (22). In the future, we may have more information about how to assess RA patients for potential responsiveness to dietary interventions in a manner that is both culturally sensitive and economically feasible.

Kitchen Spices and Rheumatoid Arthritis

The potential use for common kitchen spices with anti-inflammatory properties can be an easy and approachable dietary intervention for patients with RA that does not require a significant change in either lifestyle or food consumption patterns. Furthermore, a handful of RCTs provide evidence to demonstrate the positive impact of specific spices on RA disease activity (Table 9.2). Appropriate daily doses of cinnamon, garlic, curcumin, saffron, and ginger have been shown to reduce inflammatory markers and disease activity scores for RA (23–30). In particular, garlic and saffron were shown to decrease markers of cellular oxidative stress (26, 27). Ginger supplementation was shown to reduce gene expression for inflammatory cytokines including NFkB (24, 29).

Intermittent Fasting and Calorie Restriction for Rheumatoid Arthritis

Prolonged fasting, in which calorie intake is limited to around 300 calories per day, reduces autoinflammatory disease activity in RA and other autoimmune diseases by limiting the inflammatory functions of neutrophils (31).

The effects of prolonged, periodic fasting for RA disease activity were previously explored in three Scandinavian RCTs. Two early trials demonstrated improvement in RA symptoms after 7 days of fasting, but these positive effects were not sustained with subsequent dietary interventions (10, 11). A later trial followed 27 patients with RA on a vegetarian diet for 1 year after the completion of a 7-day fast and demonstrated sustained improvements in subjective pain scores as well as reduced CRP and ESR throughout the entirety of the study period (9).

A modern RCT (NutriFast), attempted to compare the effectiveness of fasting followed by a plant-based diet (PBD) to the currently recommended MD for patients with RA. Participants in the fasting-plus-PBD group completed a 7-day fast at the start of the study, consuming only 300 kcal per day in the form of veggie juices and broths. RA disease activity scores were compared within and between groups at various points during the 12-week intervention. Significant improvement in disease activity scores after 3 months was noted in both groups, but there was

Table 9.2 Spice Table Graphic with Positive Outcomes in Controlled Trials

	Authors	N	Outcome	Effective Daily Dose
Cinnamon	Shishehbor, et al.	36	Decreased CRP, TNFalpha, diastolic blood pressure, and DAS28	1 teaspoon
Ginger	Aryaeian, et al.	63	Decreased gene expression of NF-kB, PPAR-y, increased POxP3 gene expression Decrease in DAS28	¾ teaspoon of ground or grated ginger
Saffron	Hamidi, et al.	66	Decrease in DAS28, ESR, CRP	1 and 1/3 teaspoon
Garlic	Moosavian, et al.	62	Decrease in ESR, CRP Increased self-reported quality of life Decreased malondialdehyde levels (measure of oxidative stress)	1/3 teaspoon
Curcumin	Amalraj, et al. & Chandran, et al.	36 & 45	Decreased ESR, CRP and DAS28	2–4 teaspoons

no significant overall difference between groups at the end of the study period. Disease activity scores improved the most within and between groups in the fasting group at the end of the 7-day fast. The fasting-plus-PBD group was also noted to have a greater reduction in total leukocyte count compared to the MD group after the first 7 days of the study that persisted throughout the entire 3-month study period, suggesting that short-term fasting has sustained effects on the immune system. Researchers concluded that prolonged fasting improves RA disease activity in the short term, but MD diets were noninferior to a vegan dietary approach in terms of potential for reducing RA disease activity (32).

Time-restricted fasting, where calorie intake is not limited directly but rather restricted to a short period, could also have potential benefits for RA patients. During the month of Ramadan, those with RA who abstained from food or drink between sunrise and sunset had significant reductions in disease activity scores as well as objective markers of inflammation. Disease activity scores and inflammation markers returned to the prefasting baseline 3.5 months after the conclusion of the Ramadan period (33). Although prolonged fasting up to 7 days and time-restricted intermittent fasting can reduce disease activity in RA patients during and immediately following the fasting period, the optimal duration and interval timing for fasting periods in a manner that is safe and sustainable for patients has not yet been established.

SYSTEMIC LUPUS ERYTHEMATOSUS

Systemic lupus erythematosus (SLE) is a heterogenous, autoimmune, autoinflammatory disorder that affects multiple organ systems. In our understanding of SLE disease pathogenesis, epigenetic phenomena triggered by environmental factors induce DNA changes in the genetically susceptible individual, triggering a cascade of downstream inflammatory activity. A well-described example of this phenomenon in SLE is the appearance of the classic malar rash that occurs when the genetically vulnerable person is exposed to UVB light. Sun rays decrease enzymatic activity of DNA methyltransferase 1, which leaves promotor regions of genes coding for inflammatory cytokines accessible for gene expression (34). Dietary patterns are a modifiable environmental factor that could potentially play a role in the generation of the inflammatory response in SLE. The potential mechanisms for this have been explored extensively in lupus-prone mice but very little in humans with SLE.

SLE Mice and Diet

Much of the data on diet and lupus disease activity comes from studies of mice that are genetically engineered to develop SLE, with characteristic lupus autoantibodies, arthritis, alopecia, skin lesions, proteinuria, and nephritis. These studies allow us to understand how dietary interventions might alter immunological processes and gene expression in SLE. However, the results from these studies cannot be used to make direct conclusions about human subjects with SLE.

Diets rich in foods that promote DNA methylation, so called "methylation foods" such as dark leafy greens, cruciferous vegetables, beet root, berries, legumes, seeds, and various spices, may decrease inflammation by reducing gene expression of inflammatory cytokines. A 2013 study showed that lupus-prone mice fed methyl-rich diets had increased DNA methylation in promoter regions of the CD40lg gene, which is implicated in the development of autoreactive B cells in SLE. Mice fed the methyl rich diet also had decreased levels of the dsDNA autoantibody compared to the lupus-prone mice on the standard diet (35). Methyl rich diets for lupus-prone mice were also shown to significantly reduce proteinuria (36).

The addition of dietary omega-3 polyunsaturated fatty acids (n-3 PUFA) in lupus-prone mice has been shown to delay the onset and decrease severity of nephritis in several experiments. A group of lupus-prone mice was fed a diet supplemented with n-3 containing fish oil or a typical diet with corn oil supplementation. The n-3 supplemented mice did not develop proteinuria during the 34 weeks of the experiment, in contrast to the other groups, in which proteinuria was detected starting at 26 weeks (37).

Other studies in autoimmune mice suggest that obesity can alter the functional responsiveness of neutrophils. Increased production of radical oxygen species and earlier onset of autoantibody production were detected in lupus prone mice that were allowed to indulge in supplemental processed foods for 90 minutes daily in addition to a standard pellet diet (38).

Calorie restriction in lupus-prone mice has shown promise in regulating disease activity. Lupus-prone mice were calorie restricted (CR) to 40% the average intake of the "ad-lib" mice groups. Calorie-restricted mice had trace proteinuria at the end of the 9-month study period, whereas mice fed "ad-lib" developed measurable proteinuria by 5 months (39). Calorie-restricted lupus-prone mice also had reduced expression of platelet derived growth factor (PDGF-A) on renal histology, which has been identified previously as a pathological element in the development of lupus nephritis (40).

Dietary Interventions in Human SLE Patients

Mice studies can only tell us so much about the practical utility of dietary and nutritional interventions in human patients with SLE. Unfortunately, there are no RCTs examining the impact of dietary patterns on SLE disease activity.

We do have survey studies that explore the association between SLE and diet. In a survey of 280 patients with SLE, self-reported adherence to a Mediterranean-style dietary pattern had an inverse relationship with SLE disease activity (41).

In a large survey of mostly female SLE patients in the UK, the majority reported an interest in using dietary interventions to improve overall health and abate SLE symptoms. Patients who made dietary changes that involved eliminating or reducing meat, gluten, and dairy consumption had the most self-reported success in terms of losing weight, increasing energy levels, and decreasing joint and muscle pain (42).

The data regarding the impact of calorie restriction and fasting in humans with SLE is limited to observational trials conducted during the Ramadan fasting period. A small study of Muslim patients with quiescent lupus showed that there was no risk for increasing disease activity during and in the 3 months following the Ramadan fasting period (43). Whether or not fasting can improve disease activity in SLE patients is not studied in RCTs.

Diet Supplement Studies and SLE

Excess omega-6 fatty acid intake (typically in the form of corn and seed oils) has proinflammatory effects on the human body, whereas omega-3 fatty acids (abundant in fish oils, algae, flax seeds, chia seeds, and walnuts) have anti-inflammatory properties (44). Fiber, a nondigestible carbohydrate component found in whole plant foods, promotes digestion, regulates blood sugar, and has been associated with a decreased risk of death from diabetes, heart disease, and colorectal cancer (45).

SLE patients have self-reported lower intakes of fiber and dietary omega-3 than healthy controls, according to one survey (46). In a Japanese population, low dietary fiber intake of less than 15 grams per day was correlated with higher risk for SLE disease activity (47). SLE patients reporting higher omega-3 intake had lower disease activity scores and reported less sleep disturbance than those with lower intake. Favorable outcomes in depression, pain, and quality of life were also observed in patients with higher omega-3 intake and lower omega-6:omega-3 consumption ratio (44).

A dietary intervention involving flaxseeds, which are rich in both omega-3 and fiber, was conducted in nine patients with biopsy-proven lupus nephritis (LN). Patients served as their own controls and were asked to consume either 15 g, 30 g, or 45 g of flaxseed per day for 4-week periods, with a 5-week washout period between dosing changes. All patients had decreased proteinuria and increased creatinine clearance during each flaxseed dosing period, but the greatest benefit was seen in patients during the 30 g-per-day (4 tablespoons) consumption period (48).

Microbiome SLE Studies

SLE patients may have a lower diversity of gut microbiome species compared to healthy controls, even with a similar macronutrient intake (49). There is evidence that introduction of a low-fat, high-fiber diet can induce positive microbiome changes such as increasing the ratio of *Firmicutes:Bacteroidetes* species in patients with SLE (50).

Overall, there is a lack of RCT data for dietary interventions in SLE. There are no formal recommendations from the ACR regarding SLE and diet, but it would be reasonable to expect that patients with SLE would benefit from a dietary intervention aimed at primary and secondary cardiovascular disease risk reduction.

SERONEGATIVE SPONDYLOARTHRITIS

The group of inflammatory arthritic diseases known as "seronegative spondylarthritis" is characterized by asymmetric, large-joint arthritis, enthesitis, inflammation of the sacroiliac joints and shared genetic immune histocompatibility complex. These disorders include psoriatic arthritis (PsA), reactive arthritis, and axial and peripheral spondylarthritis. There is an associated overlap with inflammatory bowel disease, though dietary approaches for inflammatory bowel disease are beyond the scope of this book chapter.

Dietary intervention studies for seronegative spondylarthritis is limited to observational data and retrospective assessments.

Obesity and Seronegative Spondyloarthritis

Like other rheumatic diseases, spondylarthritis is an independent risk factor for cardiovascular disease (51). PsA in particular is associated with impaired insulin sensitivity and increased risk for diabetes, with 58% of PsA patients meeting criteria for metabolic syndrome (52). Obesity has also been shown to be an independent risk factor for developing PsA, especially with BMI greater than or equal to 35.0 kg/m2 or waist-to-hip ratio > 0.8 inches (53).

Weight reduction, achieved through adherence to a very-low-calorie diet for a limited period of time followed by an individualized nutrition plan, can improve disease activity in PsA (54). In a 2-year follow-up study, participants with PsA lost an average of 16% of their original body weight at one year. At 24 months, participants gained back an average of 5 kilograms, but improvements in disease activity scores were maintained (55).

Dietary Patterns and Seronegative Spondyloarthritis

There are no RCTs exploring the impact of dietary pattern interventions on disease activity in the seronegative spondyloarthropathies. A survey of dietary intake in 144 patients with both radiographic and nonradiographic axial spondylitis demonstrated a positive correlation between disease activity and consumption of ultraprocessed foods (56). In the study, higher BMI was also associated with high disease activity scores. A previous survey of Swedish patients with radiographic axial spondylitis did not find any association between diet and peripheral disease activity, though the study did not query participants about consumption of ultraprocessed foods (57).

A recent cross-sectional observational study from Italy demonstrated an inverse association between adherence to a Mediterranean-style diet and disease activity in PsA (58). In a cohort of patients with axial spondylitis, improvement in adherence to a Mediterranean-style diet by at least 20% with regular nutritional counseling was significantly associated with decreased disease activity scores during the 6-month study period (59). In both of these studies, weight loss was not observed in patients reporting increased adherence to the Mediterranean-style diet, though lower BMI at baseline did predict likelihood of increased adherence to the dietary intervention (58, 59).

The ketogenic dietary pattern, in conjunction with weight loss, has shown benefit in improving plaque psoriasis, but there are no studies examining the effects of the ketogenic diet in patients with PsA (60).

Intermittent fasting during the month of Ramadan has been correlated with decreased disease activity in patients with axial spondylitis, though this observational study only captured 20 patients and failed to show a statistically significant decrease in ESR or CRP (61).

GOUT

Gout is a rheumatic disease with a relatively ancient history, described first by the Egyptians around 2640 B.C. Hippocrates described gout as an "arthritis of the rich" due to its observed occurrence in wealthy individuals consuming large quantities of meat and alcohol (62). Thus, dietary approaches to prevent and treat gout have been of great interest, given the early observed associations between dietary consumption patterns and presentation of the disease. In the modern era, gout is no longer considered a disease of the "rich," and it has an increased prevalence in those with higher adherence to a Western dietary pattern, full of inexpensive, ultraprocessed, and fatty foods, and lacking in sufficient quantities of fruits and vegetables (63).

Recent advancements in our understanding of immunology demonstrate that gout is an inflammatory, metabolic disease, triggered by overconsumption of dietary purines in combination with genetic polymorphisms for underexcretion and overproduction of endogenous uric acid. More recent research suggests that metabolic factors such as obesity play an important role in disease pathogenesis as well (64) (Table 9.3).

Gout and Dietary Patterns

A Dietary Approach to Stop Hypertension (DASH), which emphasizes fruits, vegetables, whole grains, low-fat dairy, and limiting meat intake to less than 6 ounces per day, has been shown to have a modest but statistically significant impact on lowering serum uric acid levels (65). The urate lowering effects of the DASH dietary pattern can be detected as early as 30 days (66). Furthermore, higher lifetime intake of fruits, vegetables, whole grains, and legumes is associated with a decreased risk for developing gout (63).

There are no studies that directly measure the impact of a Mediterranean dietary pattern on primary or secondary prevention of gout. However, in a secondary analysis of patients with moderate obesity without a previous diagnosis of gout, a restricted-calorie MD led to serum reductions of urate by 113 umol/L at six months, a very small yet statistically significant result (67).

Excess intake of dietary purines from animal sources over a 2-day period increased the risk for a subsequent gout flare almost fivefold in patients with a previous diagnosis of gout (68). A prospective study of patients without a previous diagnosis of gout also demonstrated an increased risk for developing gout in the future in those with a diet high in animal-sourced purines (typically meat and seafood). Dairy intake and purine intake from vegetable sources did not appear to increase the risk for the development of gout (69). The available data suggests that low-fat dairy consumption is associated with reduced incidence of gout and may lead to reduced serum uric acid levels (70).

Gout and Miscellaneous Foods

Sugary beverages can raise serum urate levels by 1–2 mg/dl within 2 hours of ingestion (71). Calories from high-fructose corn syrup, as well as daily consumption of sugar-sweetened beverages including soda and fruit juice, have also been associated with increased risk of the development of gout in both men and women (72–74).

Cherries, which contain high concentrations of anthocyanins with anti-inflammatory and antioxidant properties, have been proposed as a nonpharmacological remedy for gout prevention. In a survey of patients with a previous history of gout, up to three servings of cherries over 2 days decreased the risk for gout flare by 45% (75). There are multiple small studies showing an association between cherry intake and decreased serum urate levels and decreased risk for recurrent gout, though these studies lack methodological homogeneity (76).

Alcohol has been proposed as a trigger for gout by inducing reversible proximal renal tubule dysfunction and therefore decreasing uric acid excretion (77). Recent evidence suggests that alcohol use alone does not increase the risk for development of hyperuricemia or gout (78). However, in individuals with preexisting gout, alcohol has been shown to be a consistent trigger preceding episodes of gout flares (79).

Interestingly, chronic, heavy alcohol drinkers often have lower serum uric acid levels due to liver dysfunction and reduced synthesis of xanthine oxidase (80). Following cessation of alcohol use, heavy alcohol users may experience an increase in serum uric acid levels and increased risk for gout (81).

Gout and Obesity

Metabolic factors including obesity have emerged as an important risk factor for the development of gout. A recent prospective cohort study analyzing data from over 51,000 male healthcare professionals suggested that modification of dietary factors, alcohol intake, and use of diuretics do not appear to decrease the risk of gout in obese males but can reduce the risk of gout in normal-weight or overweight individuals (82). Weight loss of at least 3.5 kg showed benefit for decreasing serum uric acid and decreasing the risk for gout flares over the long term (83). Obese patients undergoing bariatric surgery may experience a paradoxical increase in serum uric acid levels in the immediate postoperative period. However, in the months following bariatric surgery, the majority of patients with

Table 9.3 Impact of Diets and Individual Foods on Urate Levels, Incident Gout, and Gout Flares (reprinted with permission)

	Among people without gout*			ACR 2020 Gout guideline dietary recommendation
	Serum urate level	Risk of incident gout	Risk of gout flares	
Diet				
DASH Diet	↓	↓	No data	No recommendation
Mediterranean Diet	↓	Not enough data	No data	No recommendation
Purine-Rich Diet	↑ (short-term)	↑	↑	Recommends limiting purine intake
Weight				
Obesity	↑	↑	No data	Conditionally recommends following a weight loss program (no specific type of program recommended)
Weight Gain	↑	↑	Not enough data	
Weight Loss	↓	↓	↓	
Individual Foods				
Alcohol	↑	↑	↑	Conditionally recommends limiting alcohol intake
Caffeine	↓	↓	No data	No recommendation
Cherries	Not enough data	Not enough data	↓	No recommendation
Dairy	↓	↓	↓	No recommendation
High-Fructose Corn Syrup	↑	↑	No data	Conditionally recommends limiting intake of high-fructose corn syrup
Omega 3 Fatty Acids	Not enough data	Not enough data	Not enough data	No recommendation
Vitamin C	No effect (people with gout); may ↓ (people without gout)	Not enough data	Not enough data	Conditional recommendation against use

* Studies in people without gout unless otherwise specified

hyperuricemia prior to weight loss are able to stop taking urate-lowering therapy due to significant reductions in serum uric acid (84).

The ACR currently conditionally recommends that patients with gout reduce alcohol intake, engage in weight loss and physical activity, and avoid "purine-rich foods."

MISCELLANEOUS RHEUMATOLOGIC DISEASES

Little is known about the genetic and environmental risk factors in the pathogenesis of Sjogren's disease. In mouse studies, a high-fat diet, in which 60% of total calories are derived from fat, induces lipid accumulation and inflammation in the lacrimal gland, decreasing tear production and mimicking the lacrimal gland dysfunction seen in Sjogren's disease (85).

Adherence to a Mediterranean diet may decrease this risk for development of Sjogren's disease, and greater adherence to a Mediterranean-style diet is associated with lower disease activity scores in patients with Sjogren's disease (86, 87).

SYSTEMIC SCLEROSIS

Systemic sclerosis, an uncommon autoimmune disease characterized by multiorgan fibrosis and vasculopathy, carries the highest mortality of the rheumatic diseases (88). Over 90% of individuals with systemic sclerosis have gastrointestinal tract involvement, which typically manifests as esophageal dysfunction (89). Around 50% of systemic sclerosis patients develop fibrosis of the gastrointestinal tract, which leads to altered gut motility, bacterial overgrowth, malabsorption, constipation, diarrhea, and, in rare cases, recurrent pseudoobstruction (88, 90).

There are no studies exploring the relationship between dietary patterns and disease outcomes in systemic sclerosis. However, nutritional factors are a major concern for systemic sclerosis patients due to the frequent incidence of malnutrition (91).

Malnutrition in Systemic Sclerosis

Although only a small minority of patients with systemic sclerosis have a body mass index (BMI) of less than 18.5, the incidence of malnutrition in patients with systemic sclerosis is upward of 62.5% when using validated malnutrition scoring systems that take into account persistent chronic inflammation and reductions in muscle mass (92, 93). Malnutrition in systemic sclerosis develops due to a combination of reduced gut peristalsis and hypomotility that leads to impaired mixing and breakdown of gastric contents and bacterial overgrowth that blunts the villous architecture of absorptive surfaces in the small intestine. Small bowel water content in systemic sclerosis patients mirrors that of the malabsorptive condition celiac disease, highlighting the propensity for developing nutritional deficiencies (94). Lactose and fructose malabsorption occur in nearly 40% of individuals with systemic sclerosis (95, 96). Systemic sclerosis

patients with fructose malabsorption may benefit from a diet low in fermentable oligosaccharides, disaccharides, monosaccharides, and polyols (low FODMAP diet), which can reduce symptoms of nausea, vomiting, bloating, diarrhea, and generalized abdominal pain, as demonstrated in a small case series (95, 96).

In addition to macronutrient deficiencies, gastrointestinal distress, and weight loss, malnutrition increases the risk for micronutrient deficiencies, sarcopenia, and poor quality of life (97–99). Malnutrition has also been identified as a predictor of mortality in systemic sclerosis, making routine screening measures for malnutrition an important component of the general assessment for the patient with systemic sclerosis (100). Simple, validated screening tools can be used in the clinic to assess the short-term risk for the development of malnutrition (101, 102).

Nutritional Interventions for Systemic Sclerosis

Despite the prevalence of validated screening tools allowing for early detection of malnutrition, suggestions for intervention remain sparse. A small study of 18 systemic sclerosis patients with unintentional weight loss took part in a 6-week nutritional intervention that emphasized increased protein intake and modification of food textures to increase palatability. At the end of the intervention, patients had improvements in total muscle mass, though there were no statistically significant improvements in total calories consumed or reduction in gastrointestinal symptoms (103). The majority of patients participating in this study already met criteria for being malnourished, which limits the conclusions we can draw in regards to the utility of this intervention for preventing the development of malnutrition in at risk patients.

In the setting of severe gastrointestinal dysmotility and intolerance to enteral nutrition, parenteral nutrition (PN) can be utilized to safely provide the malnourished systemic sclerosis patient with macro- and micronutrient support (104). Unfortunately, patients with systemic sclerosis receiving PN have worse overall survival compared to patients receiving PN for an underlying diagnosis of inflammatory bowel disease (105). Although BMI and quality of life can improve with PN, the association of PN and increased mortality in systemic sclerosis patients is typically attributed to progression of their underlying disease rather than complications from PN itself (104, 106, 107).

CONCLUSION

The role of nutrition in the pathogenesis and treatment of various rheumatologic diseases continues to be a topic of exploration and debate. For patients with rheumatoid arthritis, short-term studies of dietary interventions show a trend toward mild improvement in disease activity with vegan and Mediterranean-style diets. Prolonged fasting states may also reduce disease activity. However, study sizes are small and focus on short-term outcomes. No randomized control trials of dietary interventions have been performed for any other rheumatologic diseases including SLE and seronegative spondyloarthritis. In SLE, mouse models dominate the nutrition literature and suggest that dietary changes can impact disease activity, though these studies have not been performed in humans with SLE. Recent scholarship around gout has demonstrated that this disease is as much a systemic metabolic disease as it is a disorder of purine metabolism. The modest urate-lowering effect of dietary changes through low purine consumption and high fruit and vegetable intake (DASH diet) is undermined by the metabolic dysfunction of obesity. In the seronegative spondyloarthritis family of diseases, metabolic dysfunction correlates with worsened disease activity. Conversely, weight loss has been shown to reduce disease activity scores. In systemic sclerosis, much of the literature on diet is focused on alternatives to oral nutrition in cases of severe gastrointestinal disease involvement. Early nutritional interventions are important, as many of these patients become malnourished, which remains underrecognized and underreported due to lack of clinician awareness and underutilization of malnutrition screening tools. Parenteral nutrition is a safe feeding alternative for these malnourished systemic sclerosis patients, but its implementation is typically delayed until patients have end-stage cardiac and pulmonary organ dysfunction.

In the future, microbiome studies may elucidate new understanding of the relationship between diet and autoimmune disease. Currently, there are studies suggesting key gut microbiome differences in patients with rheumatoid arthritis compared to healthy controls (108). Commensurate increases in proinflammatory gut bacteria may precipitate rheumatologic disease flares. Overall, the influence of dietary patterns on gut microbiome is strongly implied but not proven in clinical trials of patients with disease. Short-term dietary changes, on the other hand, seem to have no impact on gut microbiome composition (109).

REFERENCES

1. Adams KM, Kohlmeier M, Zeisel SH. Nutrition education in U.S. medical schools: Latest update of a national survey. *Acad Med.* 2010 Sep;85(9):1537–42.
2. Safiri S, Kolahi AA, Hoy D et al. Global, regional and national burden of rheumatoid arthritis 1990–2017: A systematic analysis of the global burden of disease study 2017. *Ann Rheum Dis.* 2019 Nov;78(11):1463–71.
3. Martínez Steele E, Baraldi LG, Louzada ML et al. Ultra-processed foods and added sugars in the US diet: Evidence from a nationally representative cross-sectional study. *BMJ Open.* 2016 Jan 9;6(3):e009892.
4. Hatami E, Aghajani M, Pourmasoumi M et al. The relationship between animal flesh foods consumption and rheumatoid arthritis: A case-control study. *Nutr J.* 2022 Jul 30;21(1):51.
5. Hu Y, Costenbader KH, Gao X et al. Sugar-sweetened soda consumption and risk of developing rheumatoid arthritis in women. *Am J Clin Nutr.* 2014 Sep;100(3):959–67.
6. Salgado E, Bes-Rastrollo M, de Irala J et al. High sodium intake is associated with self-reported rheumatoid arthritis. *Med.* 2015 Sep;94(37):e0924.
7. Sköldstam L. Vegetarian diets and rheumatoid arthritis: Is it possible that a vegetarian diet might influence the disease? *Nord Med.* 1989;104(4):112–14, 124.
8. Hafstrom I, Ringertz B, Spangberg A et al. A vegan diet free of gluten improves the signs and symptoms of rheumatoid arthritis: The effects on arthritis correlate with a reduction in antibodies to food antigens. *Rheumatol.* 2001 Oct 1;40(10):1175–9.
9. Kjeldsen-Kragh J, Borchgrevink CF, Laerum E et al. Controlled trial of

fasting and one-year vegetarian diet in rheumatoid arthritis. *Lancet.* 1991 Oct;338(8772):899–902.

10. Sköldstam L. Preliminary reports: Fasting and vegan diet in rheumatoid arthritis. *Scand J Rheumatol.* 1986 Jan 12;15(2):219–21.

11. Sköldstam L, Larsson L, Lindström FD. Effects of fasting and lactovegetarian diet on rheumatoid arthritis. *Scand J Rheumatol.* 1979 Jan 12;8(4):249–55.

12. Nenonen MT, Helve TA, Rauma AL et al. Uncooked, lactobacilli-rich, vegan food and rheumatoid arthritis. *Rheumatol.* 1998 Mar 1;37(3):274–81.

13. Barnard ND, Levin S, Crosby L et al. A randomized, crossover trial of a nutritional intervention for rheumatoid arthritis. *Am J Lifestyle Med.* 2022 Apr 3:155982762210818.

14. de Lorgeril M, Salen P, Martin JL et al. Mediterranean diet, traditional risk factors, and the rate of cardiovascular complications after myocardial infarction. *Circulation.* 1999 Feb 16;99(6):779–85.

15. Estruch R, Ros E, Salas-Salvadó J et al. Primary prevention of cardiovascular disease with a Mediterranean diet supplemented with extra-virgin olive oil or nuts. *N Engl J Med.* 2018 Jun 21;378(25):e34.

16. Guasch-Ferré M, Willett WC. The Mediterranean diet and health: A comprehensive overview. *J Intern Med.* 2021 Sep 23;290(3):549–66.

17. Skoldstam L. An experimental study of a Mediterranean diet intervention for patients with rheumatoid arthritis. *Ann Rheum Dis.* 2003 Mar 1;62(3):208–14.

18. Vadell AK, Bärebring L, Hulander E et al. Anti-Inflammatory Diet In Rheumatoid Arthritis (ADIRA)—A randomized, controlled crossover trial indicating effects on disease activity. *Am J Clin Nutr.* 2020 Jun;111(6):1203–13.

19. García-Morales JM, Lozada-Mellado M, Hinojosa-Azaola A et al. Effect of a dynamic exercise program in combination with Mediterranean diet on quality of life in women with rheumatoid arthritis. *JCR J Clin Rheumatol.* 2020 Oct;26(7S):S116–22.

20. Fraser DA, Thoen J, Djøseland O et al. Serum levels of interleukin-6 and dehydroepiandrosterone sulphate in response to either fasting or a ketogenic diet in rheumatoid arthritis patients. *Clin Exp Rheumatol.* 2000;18(3):357–62.

21. Fraser DA, Thoen J, Bondhus S et al. Reduction in serum leptin and IGF-1 but preserved T-lymphocyte numbers and activation after a ketogenic diet in rheumatoid arthritis patients. *Clin Exp Rheumatol.* 2000;18(2):209–14.

22. Lopez M, Rheumatology Advisor. *ACR releases guideline summary for use of exercise, rehabilitation, and diet in RA.* 2022. https://www.rheumatologyadvisor.com/news/acr-releases-guideline-summary-for-use-of-exercise-rehabilitation-and-diet-in-ra/

23. Amalraj A, Varma K, Jacob J et al. A novel highly bioavailable curcumin formulation improves symptoms and diagnostic indicators in rheumatoid arthritis patients: A randomized, double-blind, placebo-controlled, two-dose, three-arm, and parallel-group study. *J Med Food.* 2017 Oct;20(10):1022–30.

24. Aryaeian N, Shahram F, Mahmoudi M et al. The effect of ginger supplementation on some immunity and inflammation intermediate genes expression in patients with active Rheumatoid Arthritis. *Gene.* 2019 May;698:179–85.

25. Chandran B, Goel A. A randomized, pilot study to assess the efficacy and safety of curcumin in patients with active rheumatoid arthritis. *Phytother Res.* 2012 Nov;26(11):1719–25.

26. Hamidi Z, Aryaeian N, Abolghasemi J et al. The effect of saffron supplement on clinical outcomes and metabolic profiles in patients with active rheumatoid arthritis: A randomized, double-blind, placebo-controlled clinical trial. *Phytother Res.* 2020 Jul 11;34(7):1650–8.

27. Moosavian SP, Paknahad Z, Habibagahi Z. A randomized, double-blind, placebo-controlled clinical trial, evaluating the garlic supplement effects on some serum biomarkers of oxidative stress, and quality of life in women with rheumatoid arthritis. *Int J Clin Pract.* 2020 Jul 9;74(7).

28. Moosavian SP, Paknahad Z, Habibagahi Z et al. The effects of garlic (allium sativum) supplementation on inflammatory biomarkers, fatigue, and clinical symptoms in patients with active rheumatoid arthritis: A randomized, double-blind, placebo-controlled trial. *Phytother Res.* 2020 Nov;34(11):2953–62.

29. Aryaeian N, Mahmoudi M, Shahram F et al. The effects of ginger supplementation on IL2, TNFalpha, and IL1B cytokines gene expression levels in patients with active rheumatoid arthritis: A randomized controlled trial. *Med J Islam Repub Iran.* 2019 Dec 27;33(154).

30. Shishehbor F, Rezaeyan Safar M, Rajaei E et al. Cinnamon consumption improves clinical symptoms and inflammatory markers in women with rheumatoid arthritis. *J Am Coll Nutr.* 2018 Nov 17;37(8):685–90.

31. Hafström I, Ringertz B, Gyllenhammar H et al. Effects of fasting on disease activity, neutrophil function, fatty acid composition, and leukotriene biosynthesis in patients with rheumatoid arthritis. *Arthritis Rheum.* 1988 May;31(5):585–92.

32. Hartmann AM, Dell'Oro M, Spoo M et al. To eat or not to eat—An exploratory randomized controlled trial on fasting and plant-based diet in rheumatoid arthritis (NutriFast-study). *Front Nutr.* 2022 Nov 2;9.

33. Ben Nessib D, Maatallah K, Ferjani H et al. Sustainable positive effects of Ramadan intermittent fasting in rheumatoid arthritis. *Clin Rheumatol.* 2022 Feb 10;41(2):399–403.

34. Nawrocki MJ, Majewski D, Puszczewicz M et al. Decreased mRNA expression levels of DNA methyltransferases type 1 and 3A in systemic lupus erythematosus. *Rheumatol Int.* 2017 May 27;37(5):775–83.

35. Strickland FM, Hewagama A, Wu A et al. Diet influences expression of autoimmune-associated genes and disease severity by epigenetic mechanisms in a transgenic mouse model of lupus. *Arthritis Rheum.* 2013 Jul;65(7):1872–81.

36. Nikolova-Ganeva K, Bradyanova S, Manoylov I et al. Methyl-rich diet ameliorates lupus-like disease in MRL/lpr mice. *Immunobiol.* 2022 Nov;227(6):152282.

37. Pestka JJ, Vines LL, Bates MA et al. Comparative effects of n-3, n-6 and n-9 unsaturated fatty acid-rich diet consumption on lupus nephritis, autoantibody production and CD4+ T cell-related gene responses in the autoimmune NZBWF1 mouse. *PLoS One.* 2014 Jun 19;9(6):e100255.

38. Toller-Kawahisa JE, Canicoba NC, Venancio VP et al. Systemic lupus erythematosus onset in lupus-prone B6.MRL/lpr mice is influenced by weight gain and is preceded by an increase in neutrophil oxidative burst activity. *Free Radic Biol Med.* 2015 Sep;86:362–73.

39. Reddy Avula CP, Lawrence RA, Zaman K et al. Inhibition of intracellular peroxides and apoptosis of lymphocytes in lupus-prone B/W mice by dietary n-6 and n-3 lipids with calorie restriction. *J Clin Immunol.* 2002;22(4):206–19.

40. Troyer DA, Chandrasekar B, Barnes JL et al. Calorie restriction decreases Platelet-Derived Growth Factor (PDGF)-a and thrombin receptor mRNA expression in autoimmune murine lupus nephritis. *Clin Exp Immunol.* 2003 Oct 29;108(1):58–62.

41. Pocovi-Gerardino G, Correa-Rodríguez M, Callejas-Rubio JL et al. Beneficial effect of Mediterranean diet on disease activity and cardiovascular risk in systemic lupus erythematosus patients: A cross-sectional study. *Rheumatol.* 2021 Jan 5;60(1):160–9.

42. Knippenberg A, Robinson GA, Wincup C et al. Plant-based dietary changes may improve symptoms in patients with systemic lupus erythematosus. *Lupus.* 2022 Jan 3;31(1):65–76.

43. Goharifar H, Faezi ST, Paragomi P et al. The effect of Ramadan fasting on quiescent Systemic Lupus Erythematosus (SLE) patients' disease activity, health quality of life and lipid profile: A pilot study. *Rheumatol Int.* 2015 Aug 14;35(8):1409–14.

44. Charoenwoodhipong P, Harlow SD, Marder W et al. Dietary omega polyunsaturated fatty acid intake and patient-reported outcomes in systemic lupus erythematosus: The Michigan lupus epidemiology and surveillance program. *Arthritis Care Res* (Hoboken). 2020 Jul 29;72(7):874–81.

45. Reynolds A, Mann J, Cummings J et al. Carbohydrate quality and human health:

A series of systematic reviews and meta-analyses. *Lancet*. 2019 Feb;393(10170):434–45.

46. Elkan AC, Anania C, Gustafsson T et al. Diet and fatty acid pattern among patients with SLE: Associations with disease activity, blood lipids and atherosclerosis. *Lupus*. 2012 Nov 28;21(13):1405–11.

47. Minami Y, Hirabayashi Y, Nagata C et al. Intakes of vitamin B6 and dietary fiber and clinical course of systemic lupus erythematosus: A prospective study of Japanese female patients. *J Epidemiol*. 2011;21(4):246–54.

48. Clark WF, Parbtani A, Huff MW et al. Flaxseed: A potential treatment for lupus nephritis. *Kidney Int*. 1995 Aug;48(2):475–80.

49. van der Meulen TA, Harmsen HJM, Vila AV et al. Shared gut, but distinct oral microbiota composition in primary Sjögren's syndrome and systemic lupus erythematosus. *J Autoimmun*. 2019 Feb;97:77–87.

50. Hevia A, Milani C, López P et al. Intestinal dysbiosis associated with systemic lupus erythematosus. *mBio*. 2014 Oct 31;5(5).

51. Papagoras C, Voulgari PV, Drosos AA. Atherosclerosis and cardiovascular disease in the spondyloarthritides, particularly ankylosing spondylitis and psoriatic arthritis. *Clin Exp Rheumatol*. 2013;31(4):612–20.

52. Raychaudhuri SK, Chatterjee S, Nguyen C et al. Increased prevalence of the metabolic syndrome in patients with psoriatic arthritis. *Metab Syndr Relat Disord*. 2010 Aug;8(4):331–4.

53. Li W, Han J, Qureshi AA. Obesity and risk of incident psoriatic arthritis in US women. *Ann Rheum Dis*. 2012 Aug;71(8):1267–72.

54. Klingberg E, Bilberg A, Björkman S et al. Weight loss improves disease activity in patients with psoriatic arthritis and obesity: An interventional study. *Arthritis Res Ther*. 2019 Dec 11;21(1):17.

55. Klingberg E, Björkman S, Eliasson B et al. Weight loss is associated with sustained improvement of disease activity and cardiovascular risk factors in patients with psoriatic arthritis and obesity: A prospective intervention study with two years of follow-up. *Arthritis Res Ther*. 2020 Dec 22;22(1):254.

56. Vergne-Salle P, Salle L, Fressinaud-Marie AC et al. Diet and disease activity in patients with axial spondyloarthritis: Spondyloarthritis and NUTrition study (SANUT). *Nutrients*. 2022 Nov 9;14(22):4730.

57. Sundström B, Wållberg-Jonsson S, Johansson G. Diet, disease activity, and gastrointestinal symptoms in patients with ankylosing spondylitis. *Clin Rheumatol*. 2011 Jan 27;30(1):71–6.

58. Caso F, Navarini L, Carubbi F et al. Mediterranean diet and psoriatic arthritis activity: A multicenter cross-sectional study. *Rheumatol Int*. 2020 Jun 11;40(6):951–8.

59. Ometto F, Ortolan A, Farber D et al. Mediterranean diet in axial spondyloarthritis: An observational study in an Italian monocentric cohort. *Arthritis Res Ther*. 2021 Dec 20;23(1):219.

60. Castaldo G, Pagano I, Grimaldi M et al. Effect of very-low-calorie ketogenic diet on psoriasis patients: A nuclear magnetic resonance-based metabolomic study. *J Proteome Res*. 2021 Mar 5;20(3):1509–21.

61. Ben Nessib D, Maatallah K, Ferjani H et al. Impact of Ramadan diurnal intermittent fasting on rheumatic diseases. *Clin Rheumatol*. 2020 Aug 5;39(8):2433–40.

62. Nuki G, Simkin PA. A concise history of gout and hyperuricemia and their treatment. *Arthritis Res Ther*. 2006;8(Suppl 1):S1.

63. Rai SK, Fung TT, Lu N et al. The Dietary Approaches to Stop Hypertension (DASH) diet, Western diet, and risk of gout in men: Prospective cohort study. *BMJ*. 2017 May 9;j1794.

64. Danve A, Sehra ST, Neogi T. Role of diet in hyperuricemia and gout. *Best Pract Res Clin Rheumatol*. 2021 Dec;35(4):101723.

65. Juraschek SP, Yokose C, McCormick N et al. Effects of dietary patterns on serum urate: Results from a randomized trial of the effects of diet on hypertension. *Arthritis Rheumatol*. 2021 Jun 23;73(6):1014–20.

66. Tang O, Miller ER, Gelber AC et al. Dash diet and change in serum uric acid over time. *Clin Rheumatol*. 2017 Jun 31;36(6):1413–17.

67. Yokose C, McCormick N, Rai SK et al. Effects of low-fat, Mediterranean, or low-carbohydrate weight loss diets on

serum urate and cardiometabolic risk factors: A secondary analysis of the Dietary Intervention Randomized Controlled Trial (DIRECT). *Diabetes Care.* 2020 Nov 1;43(11):2812–20.

68. Zhang Y, Chen C, Choi H et al. Purine-rich foods intake and recurrent gout attacks. *Ann Rheum Dis.* 2012 Sep;71(9):1448–53.

69. Choi HK, Atkinson K, Karlson EW et al. Purine-rich foods, dairy and protein intake, and the risk of gout in men. *N Engl J Med.* 2004 Mar 11;350(11):1093–103.

70. Dalbeth N, Palmano K. Effects of dairy intake on hyperuricemia and gout. *Curr Rheumatol Rep.* 2011 Apr;13(2):132–7.

71. Stirpe F, Della CE, Bonetti E et al. Fructose-induced Hyperuricæmia. *Lancet.* 1970 Dec;296(7686):1310–11.

72. Choi HK, Willett W, Curhan G. Fructose-rich beverages and risk of gout in women. *JAMA.* 2010 Nov 24;304(20):2270–8.

73. Choi HK, Curhan G. Soft drinks, fructose consumption, and the risk of gout in men: Prospective cohort study. *BMJ.* 2008 Feb 9;336(7639):309–12.

74. Choi JWJ, Ford ES, Gao X et al. Sugar-sweetened soft drinks, diet soft drinks, and serum uric acid level: The third national health and nutrition examination survey. *Arthritis Rheum.* 2008 Jan;59(1):109–16.

75. Zhang Y, Neogi T, Chen C et al. Cherry consumption and decreased risk of recurrent gout attacks. *Arthritis Rheum.* 2012 Dec;64(12):4004–11.

76. Chen PE, Liu CY, Chien WH et al. Effectiveness of cherries in reducing uric acid and gout: A systematic review. *Evid Based Complement Alternat Med.* 2019;2019:9896757.

77. De Marchi S, Cecchin E, Basile A et al. Renal tubular dysfunction in chronic alcohol abuse—Effects of abstinence. *N Engl J Med.* 1993 Dec 23;329(26):1927–34.

78. Syed AAS, Fahira A, Yang Q et al. The relationship between alcohol consumption and gout: A mendelian randomization study. *Genes* (Basel). 2022 Mar 22;13(4).

79. Nieradko-Iwanicka B. The role of alcohol consumption in pathogenesis of gout. *Crit Rev Food Sci Nutr.* 2022;62(25):7129–37.

80. Decaux G, Dumont I, Naeije N et al. High uric acid and urea clearance in cirrhosis secondary to increased "effective vascular volume". *Am J Med.* 1982 Sep;73(3):328–34.

81. Liberopoulos EN, Miltiadous GA, Elisaf MS. Alcohol intake, serum uric acid concentrations, and risk of gout. *Lancet.* 2004 Jul;364(9430):246–7.

82. McCormick N, Rai SK, Lu N et al. Estimation of primary prevention of gout in men through modification of obesity and other key lifestyle factors. *JAMA Netw Open.* 2020 Nov 2;3(11):e2027421.

83. Nielsen SM, Bartels EM, Henriksen M et al. Weight loss for overweight and obese individuals with gout: A systematic review of longitudinal studies. *Ann Rheum Dis.* 2017 Nov;76(11):1870–82.

84. Dalbeth N, Chen P, White M et al. Impact of bariatric surgery on serum urate targets in people with morbid obesity and diabetes: A prospective longitudinal study. *Ann Rheum Dis.* 2014 May;73(5):797–802.

85. He X, Zhao Z, Wang S et al. High-fat diet—Induced functional and pathologic changes in lacrimal gland. *Am J Pathol.* 2020 Dec;190(12):2387–402.

86. Carubbi F, Alunno A, Mai F et al. Adherence to the Mediterranean diet and the impact on clinical features in primary Sjögren's syndrome. *Clin Exp Rheumatol.* 2021;39(Suppl 133, 6):190–6.

87. Machowicz A, Hall I, de Pablo P et al. Mediterranean diet and risk of Sjögren's syndrome. *Clin Exp Rheumatol.* 2020;38 Suppl 126(4):216–21.

88. Volkmann ER, Andréasson K, Smith V. Systemic sclerosis. *Lancet.* 2023 Jan 28;401(10373):304–18.

89. McMahan ZH. Gastrointestinal involvement in systemic sclerosis: An update. *Curr Opin Rheumatol* [Internet]. 2019 Nov;31(6):561–8. www.ncbi.nlm.nih.gov/pubmed/31389815

90. Steen VD, Medsger TA. Severe organ involvement in systemic sclerosis with diffuse scleroderma. *Arthritis Rheum.* 2000 Nov;43(11):2437–44.

91. Burlui AM, Cardoneanu A, Macovei LA et al. Diet in scleroderma: Is there a need for intervention? *Diagnostics* (Basel). 2021 Nov 15;11(11).

92. Rosato E, Gigante A, Gasperini ML et al. Assessing malnutrition in systemic sclerosis with global leadership initiative on malnutrition and European society of clinical nutrition and metabolism criteria. *JPEN J Parenter Enteral Nutr.* 2021 Mar;45(3):618–24.

93. Wojteczek A, Dardzińska JA, Małgorzewicz S et al. Prevalence of malnutrition in systemic sclerosis patients assessed by different diagnostic tools. *Clin Rheumatol.* 2020 Jan;39(1):227–32.

94. Lam C, Sanders DS, Lanyon P et al. Increased fasting small-bowel water content in untreated coeliac disease and scleroderma as assessed by magnetic resonance imaging. *United European Gastroenterol J.* 2019 Dec;7(10):1353–60.

95. Marie I, Leroi AM, Gourcerol G et al. Fructose malabsorption in systemic sclerosis. *Med.* 2015 Sep;94(39):e1601.

96. Marie I, Leroi AM, Gourcerol G et al. Lactose malabsorption in systemic sclerosis. *Aliment Pharmacol Ther.* 2016 Nov;44(10):1123–33.

97. Caimmi C, Caramaschi P, Venturini A et al. Malnutrition and sarcopenia in a large cohort of patients with systemic sclerosis. *Clin Rheumatol.* 2018 Apr;37(4):987–97.

98. Dupont R, Longué M, Galinier A et al. Impact of micronutrient deficiency & malnutrition in systemic sclerosis: Cohort study and literature review. *Autoimmun Rev.* 2018 Nov;17(11):1081–9.

99. Preis E, Franz K, Siegert E et al. The impact of malnutrition on quality of life in patients with systemic sclerosis. *Eur J Clin Nutr.* 2018 Apr;72(4):504–10.

100. Cruz-Domínguez MP, García-Collinot G, Saavedra MA et al. Malnutrition is an independent risk factor for mortality in Mexican patients with systemic sclerosis: A cohort study. *Rheumatol Int.* 2017 Jul;37(7):1101–9.

101. Bagnato G, Pigatto E, Bitto A et al. The PREdictor of MAlnutrition in Systemic Sclerosis (PREMASS) score: A combined index to predict 12 months onset of malnutrition in systemic sclerosis. *Front Med* (Lausanne). 2021;8:651748.

102. Hvas CL, Harrison E, Eriksen MK et al. Nutritional status and predictors of weight loss in patients with systemic sclerosis. *Clin Nutr ESPEN.* 2020 Dec;40:164–70.

103. Doerfler B, Allen TS, Southwood C et al. Medical Nutrition Therapy for Patients with Advanced Systemic Sclerosis (MNT PASS): A pilot intervention study. *JPEN J Parenter Enteral Nutr.* 2017 May;41(4):678–84.

104. Harrison E, Herrick AL, McLaughlin J et al. 22 years experience managing patients with systemic sclerosis on home parenteral nutrition. *Clin Nutr ESPEN.* 2015 Oct;10(5):e178.

105. Dibb M, Soop M, Teubner A et al. Survival and nutritional dependence on home parenteral nutrition: Three decades of experience from a single referral centre. *Clin Nutr.* 2017 Apr;36(2):570–6.

106. Jawa H, Fernandes G, Saqui O et al. Home parenteral nutrition in patients with systemic sclerosis: A retrospective review of 12 cases. *J Rheumatol.* 2012 May;39(5):1004–7.

107. Stanga Z, Aeberhard C, Schärer P et al. Home parenteral nutrition is beneficial in systemic sclerosis patients with gastrointestinal dysfunction. *Scand J Rheumatol.* 2016 Jan;45(1):32–5.

108. Yu D, Du J, Pu X et al. The gut microbiome and metabolites are altered and interrelated in patients with rheumatoid arthritis. *Front Cell Infect Microbiol.* 2021;11:763507.

109. Coras R, Martino C, Gauglitz JM et al. Baseline microbiome and metabolome are associated with response to ITIS diet in an exploratory trial in patients with rheumatoid arthritis. *Clin Transl Med.* 2022 Jul 8;12(7).

10

Gastroenterological Considerations for Patients on Rheumatologic Medications

MOHAMAD KHALED ALMUJARKESH, SHUBHA BHAT, AND JAMI KINNUCAN

INTRODUCTION

Rheumatologic conditions are often treated using medications such as conventional DMARDs, including methotrexate (MTX), azathioprine, sulfasalazine, hydroxychloroquine (HCQ), and leflunomide or biologic DMARDs, including rituximab, etanercept, tumor necrosis factor (TNF) inhibitors, interleukin-1 and -6 inhibitors, and other anticytokine therapies. Additionally, adjunctive medications such as nonsteroidal anti-inflammatories (NSAIDs) and glucocorticoids are often utilized.

Adverse events were reported as the most frequent cause of medication discontinuation in patients taking DMARDs (1). The anti-inflammatory and immunosuppressive nature of these medications has been known to cause several multisystem side effects, with gastrointestinal (GI)-related adverse effects being the most common among DMARDs (1). Adverse GI effects can range from mild symptoms of nausea and vomiting to more severe conditions such as perforation or enteritis. Studies have shown when adjusted for demographics such as age and sex, patients on immunosuppressive therapy have a higher incidence of GI adverse effects (1). For some of the GI adverse effects that are seen more commonly with

certain rheumatologic therapies, adjuvant therapies may be recommended to prevent undesired symptoms. Thus, to minimize treatment nonadherence and optimize treatment outcomes and safety, it is important for clinicians to be aware of potential medication adverse effects and provide prompt evaluation and management.

COMMON GI SYMPTOMS RESULTING FROM RHEUMATOLOGIC MEDICATIONS

Nausea and Vomiting

Nausea and vomiting are some of the most common medication-induced adverse effects. These symptoms are most often observed with MTX treatment, with 42% of patients with rheumatoid arthritis endorsing primarily nausea and/or vomiting (~3.9%) within 12 months of use (2). Mechanisms for MTX-induced nausea and vomiting may be due to its direct mechanism of inhibiting the proliferation of healthy cells, folic acid deficiency, or possible anticipation of expecting adverse effects with treatment. A methotrexate intolerance severity score (MISS) has been established to assess for GI intolerances with this treatment and is commonly used for patients with juvenile idiopathic arthritis,

DOI: 10.1201/9781003367307-10

rheumatoid arthritis, or psoriatic arthritis. MISS is a 12-item questionnaire that assesses for symptoms of abdominal pain, nausea, vomiting, and behavioral changes with consideration of MTX timing and symptom severity. Timing of MTX-associated nausea and vomiting includes prior to taking (anticipatory), after, or when thinking of taking MTX (associative). Symptom severity is graded on a scale of none, mild, moderate, or severe. Scores range from 0 to 36, with a score of 6 or higher being indicative of methotrexate intolerance if at least 1 point is from the anticipatory, behavioral, or associative categories (3).

Early identification of MTX intolerance using this scale can assist with appropriate medication changes to help improve patient adherence. Nausea and/or vomiting (23%) can also be seen with azathioprine use. Sulfasalazine and leflunomide are some of the other rheumatologic medications that can be associated with nausea and vomiting, but this is to a lesser degree than the former agents discussed.

Enteritis with or without Gastrointestinal Bleeding

NSAIDs and corticosteroids are often used in patients with rheumatologic conditions to provide acute anti-inflammatory and symptomatic relief. NSAIDs cause gastric and duodenal irritation through a mechanism of nonselective COX inhibition, which leads to prostaglandin deficiency, resulting in hypermotility and microvascular changes, which, in turn, causes gastric or duodenal inflammation (4). Patients with frequent NSAID use have a 2.5- to 5-fold increase in the risk of GI complications compared to those not taking NSAIDs (5). Mucosal injury can result in erosion and, in severe cases, progress to ulcers and perforations. Patients who take corticosteroids in addition to NSAIDs are at a greater increased risk of mucosal disruption. The risk of GI bleed-related events has been observed with corticosteroid monotherapy and increases 4-fold when combined with NSAID use. MTX has also been implicated in causing mucosal disruption (6).

Medication-Induced Colitis

Microscopic colitis is a condition involving inflammation of the colon that is associated with histologic changes and is often characterized as lymphocytic or collagenous colitis. Patients often present with watery nonbloody diarrhea, with also some experiencing urgency and nocturnal episodes of bowel movements. Chronic NSAID use has been associated with a 4-fold increase of developing microscopic colitis. TNF inhibitors have also been found to be associated with drug-induced colitis per reported cases involving the use of infliximab, etanercept, certolizumab, and adalimumab. These agents may cause de novo colitis or worsen existing colitis. Endoscopic and histologic patterns included mucosal erosions, ulcerations, and endothelial apoptosis and may mimic ulcerative colitis (7). A Danish study found a 2-fold increased risk of developing Crohn's disease or ulcerative colitis in those taking TNF inhibitors for autoimmune pathologies excluding inflammatory bowel disease (8).

Diarrhea

Diarrhea is one of the most reported adverse effects of DMARDs, including sulfasalazine, leflunomide, and HCQ. Pathophysiology of diarrhea ranges from drug-induced colitis to mild nonspecific inflammation. HCQ's most common adverse reactions are GI related, including anorexia, nausea, and diarrhea, which usually are reported within the first few weeks of initiation (9). Symptoms typically resolve with dose reduction or discontinuation of therapy.

Pancreatitis

Drug-induced pancreatitis is usually self-limited with a good prognosis. Azathioprine and 6-mercaptopurine (6MP) have been associated with increased risk for pancreatitis (3–4%) (10). Pancreatitis in patients with rheumatoid arthritis treated with azathioprine or 6MP is rare but has been reported (11). Pancreatitis occurs more commonly with azathioprine than 6MP. The ideal recommendation is to discontinue the offending agent, but, in some cases, since these two medications both work to inhibit purine synthesis, azathioprine can be switched to 6MP or vice versa. These adjustments are to be made on an individual basis only and are not generalizable, as individual responses can vary (12). Additionally, combination medication (typically adding azathioprine to a biologic therapy) for rheumatoid arthritis can further increase this risk for pancreatitis in some patients.

Hepatotoxicity

DMARD therapies can be associated with hepatotoxicity, some of which have been cumulative dose effects such as MTX and azathioprine. Hepatotoxic effects include the development of drug-induced liver injury (DILI) and autoimmune hepatitis. NSAIDs and sulfasalazine have been associated with both hepatocellular and cholestatic injury patterns. Conversely, leflunomide-associated injury is hepatocellular, while azathioprine is mixed (13). MTX and sulfasalazine have been associated with chronic DILI. Several TNF inhibitors (etanercept, adalimumab, and infliximab) have also been associated with DILI. Although both cholestatic and hepatocellular injury patterns have been reported, hepatocellular is the most predominant type with evidence of autoimmune characteristics. While there is no specific threshold, suspicions of DILI should arise when there is a 3-fold or higher rise in baseline AST/ALT. Medication exposure timing and other causes should be considered prior to making a diagnosis of DILI (14).

For many of these therapies, it is recommended to obtain and monitor liver function tests at baseline and after initiation or dose adjustment. Hepatoxicity has been reported in monotherapy and with combination therapy (addition of immunomodulator to other DMARDs therapy). While patients may tolerate a single agent, they may experience hepatotoxicity with combination therapy. Patients with a concomitant history of alcohol use, autoimmune hepatitis, steatohepatitis, and viral hepatitis have an increased risk of hepatotoxicity with the use of MTX (15, 16).

Viral Hepatitis

The immunosuppressive nature of rheumatologic medications additionally renders patients prone to infections. Most DMARDs, therefore, require hepatitis screening prior to initiation. Screening for hepatitis B includes assessment for immunity, active infection, or past infection. For those without immunity, recommendations to receive immunizations are appropriate. In individuals with active infection, prompt referral to hepatology and initiation of antiviral therapy is often indicated. Patients with prior hepatitis B infection (hepatitis B core antibody positive) are at risk for reactivation with initiation of certain higher-risk immunosuppressive therapies. Current guidelines recommend the use of prophylaxis for those patients taking medications with the highest risk of reactivation (> 10%), including rituximab and high-dose corticosteroids. Drugs with a moderate risk of reactivation (1% to 10%) include TNF inhibitors (infliximab, etanercept, adalimumab), tyrosine kinase, and cytokine inhibitors (17). Reactivation of hepatitis B in these immunosuppressed individuals can be catastrophic, leading to fulminant liver failure and even death. Thus, initial and ongoing assessment as it relates to immunosuppressive therapy is critical.

PREVENTION AND TREATMENT OF GI MANIFESTATIONS

Clinician awareness and patient education are important first steps to preventing undesirable adverse effects. It is important for clinicians to assess a patient's risk for possible adverse effects prior to initiating any therapy (Table 10.1). For example, patients on antiplatelet or anticoagulant medications, with concomitant liver dysfunction, and/or over the age of 60 years have a higher risk of NSAID-induced GI bleed. Compared to histamine (H2) blockers, proton pump inhibitors (PPIs) have been shown to reduce the risk of gastroduodenal toxicity. Thus, PPIs are indicated in patients taking NSAIDs along with corticosteroids to reduce the risk of GI bleed. Alternatively, use of selective COX inhibitors may be favored, given the lower risk of GI bleed when compared to other NSAID therapies utilizing a nonselective mechanism (18).

MTX-associated nausea and vomiting can be mitigated with adjuvant antiemetic therapy and/or H2 blockers. Patients taking folic acid supplementation while on chronic MTX have been shown to have decreased adverse effects, including nausea, hepatotoxicity, and stomatitis. Leucovorin (folinic acid) can be used as an alternate to folic acid. For azathioprine or 6MP, splitting doses (a.m. and p.m.) can mitigate these undesirable effects. Variations in the timing of HCQ by taking doses

Table 10.1 GI Considerations and Preventive Strategies for Rheumatologic Drugs

Drug	Common GI side effects	Prevention/treatment considerations
Azathioprine	Nausea/vomiting (23%), pancreatitis (3.3%), DILI, elevated LFTs (5%)	Split dose, medication change to 6MP, dose reduction, premedication
Methotrexate (MTX)	Nausea (20% to 30%), diarrhea (15%), elevated LFTs (14.1%), liver fibrosis (5%)	Folic acid supplementation, leucovorin rescue, antiemetics, H2 blockers, monitoring liver enzymes
Sulfasalazine	Nausea (19%), diarrhea, abdominal pain (8%), DILI (frequency not defined), abnormal hepatic function tests 4%)	Hydration, antiemetics, dose reduction, can impair MTX renal clearance, enteric coated form
Leflunomide	Diarrhea (22% to 27%), nausea (13%), hepatotoxicity (1–4%)	Cholestyramine washout in toxicity, gradual dose titration, monitoring liver enzymes
Hydroxychloroquine (HCQ)	Abdominal pain/diarrhea (22.7%)	Gradual titration, antiemetics
TNF inhibitors	Infliximab hepatotoxicity (8.3%), autoimmune hepatitis (case reports)	LFT monitoring, corticosteroids, medication cessation
Rituximab	Reactivation of HBV (20% to 55% in HBsAg+ patients and 3% in HBsAg- patients)	Screening for HBV exposure, HBV prophylaxis
NSAID	Nausea, gastritis (60% to 70%), peptic ulcer disease (30% to 40%), GI bleeding (30%)	PPI, limit dose/exposure, selective COX inhibitor
Corticosteroids	GI bleeding (2.3%), perforation, pancreatitis (0.1–2%), may increase the risk of gastrointestinal bleeding or perforation by 40%	PPI indicated with concomitant NSAID use

DILI: drug-induced liver injury

at bedtime may improve symptoms. Furthermore, gradually titrating dosing over a period of days may decrease initial side effects. These additional mitigation opportunities have shown to reduce symptoms and ultimately improve medication adherence.

Drug-induced enteritis management is generally supportive. The offending agent must be identified and stopped. Due to diarrhea and subsequent volume loss from enteritis, hydration must be encouraged, and if required, IV fluids can be administered. To mitigate symptoms, antidiarrheal agents may be used with caution, as these agents may delay clearance of the offending agent. In severe cases of drug-induced

enteritis, corticosteroid short course can provide benefit in decreasing inflammatory burden and symptoms (19).

It is important to be aware of the different patterns of hepatotoxicity caused by individual agents and to exclude other causes. Monitoring of liver enzymes and albumin is necessary in certain medications such as MTX. If there is an increase in enzyme levels, a thorough history must be obtained for exposure of any additional hepatotoxic causes such as alcohol, NSAIDs, or viral hepatitis. If no other cause is identified and levels remain elevated, reducing the dose of or discontinuing the potential offending medication should be considered.

CONCLUSION

Management of most rheumatologic conditions consists of targeted inflammatory control with early initiation of treatment and medication optimization. Due to the chronic nature of rheumatologic conditions, medications are routinely administered for prolonged periods of time and may result in GI-related adverse effects. Given the importance of medication adherence to achieve optimal disease outcomes and the most common cause of medication discontinuation being related to adverse effects, it is important for clinicians to anticipate, educate patients about, and manage these adverse effects in order to help optimize medication adherence and outcomes.

REFERENCES

1. Aletaha D, Kapral T, Smolen JS. Toxicity profiles of traditional disease modifying antirheumatic drugs for rheumatoid arthritis. *Ann Rheum Dis*. 2003 May;62(5):482–6. PMC1754550
2. Sherbini AA, Gwinnutt JM, Hyrich KL et al. Rates and predictors of methotrexate-related adverse events in patients with early rheumatoid arthritis: Results from a nationwide UK study. *Rheumatol* (Oxford). 2022 Oct 6;61(10):3930–8. PMC9536779
3. Amaral JM, Brito MJM, Kakehasi AM. High frequency of methotrexate intolerance in longstanding rheumatoid arthritis: Using the methotrexate intolerance severity score (MISS). *Adv Rheumatol*. 2020 Aug 26;60(1):43. PMID: 32843102
4. Takeuchi K. Pathogenesis of NSAID-induced gastric damage: Importance of cyclooxygenase inhibition and gastric hypermotility. *World J Gastroenterol*. 2012 May 14;18(18):2147–60. PMC3351764
5. Arroyo M, Lanas A. NSAIDs-induced gastrointestinal damage: Review. *Minerva Gastroenterol Dietol*. 2006 Sep;52(3):249–59. PMID: 16971869
6. Troeltzsch M, von Blohn G, Kriegelstein S et al. Oral mucositis in patients receiving low-dose methotrexate therapy for rheumatoid arthritis: Report of 2 cases and literature review. *Oral Surg Oral Med Oral Pathol Oral Radiol*. 2013 May;115(5):e28–33. PMC6632433
7. Hamdeh S, Micic D, Hanauer S. Drug-induced colitis. *Clin Gastroenterol Hepatol*. 2021 Sep;19(9):1759–79. PMID: 32360808
8. Korzenik J, Larsen MD, Nielsen J et al. Increased risk of developing Crohn's disease or ulcerative colitis in 17018 patients while under treatment with anti-TNFα agents, particularly etanercept, for autoimmune diseases other than inflammatory bowel disease. *Aliment Pharmacol Ther*. 2019 Aug;50(3):289–94. PMID: 31267570
9. Munster T, Gibbs JP, Shen D et al. Hydroxychloroquine concentration-response relationships in patients with rheumatoid arthritis. *Arthritis Rheum*. 2002 Jun;46(6):1460–9. PMID: 12115175
10. Nitsche CJ, Jamieson N, Lerch MM et al. Drug induced pancreatitis. *Best Pract Res Clin Gastroenterol*. 2010 Apr;24(2):143–55. PMID: 20227028
11. Chang CC, Chiou CS, Lin HL et al. Increased risk of acute pancreatitis in patients with rheumatoid arthritis: A population-based cohort study. *PLoS One*. 2015 Aug 11;10(8):e0135187. PMC4532490
12. Gordon M, Grafton-Clarke C, Akobeng A et al. Pancreatitis associated with azathioprine and 6-mercaptopurine use in Crohn's disease: A systematic review. *Frontline Gastroenterol*. 2020 Jun 11;12(5):423–36. PMC8989005
13. Aithal G. Hepatotoxicity related to anti-rheumatic drug. *Nat Rev Rheumatol*. 2011 Mar;7(3):139–50. PMID: 2126345
14. Fisher K, Vuppalanchi R, Saxena R. Drug-induced liver injury. *Arch Pathol Lab Med*. 2015 Jul;139(7):876–87. PMID: 26125428
15. FDA. *Drug safety communication: New boxed warning for severe liver injury with rthritis drug Arava (leflunomide)*. 2010. www.fda.gov/Drugs/DrugSafety/ PostmarketDrugSafetyInformationfor PatientsandProviders/ucm218679.htm
16. Kremer JM, Lee RG, Tolman KG. Liver histology in rheumatoid arthritis patients receiving long-term methotrexate therapy. A prospective study with baseline and sequential biopsy samples. *Arthritis Rheum*. 1989 Feb;32(2):121–7. PMID: 2920047

17. Fleischmann RM. Safety of biologic therapy in rheumatoid arthritis and other autoimmune diseases: Focus on rituximab. *Semin Arthritis Rheum.* 2009 Feb;38(4):265–80. PMID: 18336874

18. Feldman M, McMahon AT. Do cyclooxygenase-2 inhibitors provide benefits similar to those of traditional nonsteroidal anti-inflammatory drugs, with less gastrointestinal toxicity? *Ann Intern Med.* 2000 Jan 18;132(2):134–43. PMID: 10644275

19. Tonolini M. Acute nonsteroidal anti-inflammatory drug-induced colitis. *J Emerg Trauma Shock.* 2013 Oct;6(4):301–3. PMC3841543

11

Rheumatologic Implications for Patients on Gastrointestinal Medications

RYAN MASSAY AND SEETHA U. MONRAD

INTRODUCTION

In recent decades, many new medications have revolutionized the management of gastroenterological conditions and resulted in better disease outcomes. Since their introduction in the early 1990s, proton pump inhibitors have become the standard of care for treatment of gastric acid–related disorders. Biologic and small molecule therapies are resulting in greater rates of remission and increased quality of life for patients with inflammatory bowel disease. However, as these agents have been more frequently prescribed and over longer periods of time, there is heightened recognition of and experience with rheumatologic complications from these agents. These include adverse immunologic events such as drug-induced autoimmune disorders, effects on bone metabolism, and others. It is important for practicing rheumatologists and gastroenterologists to have a contemporary understanding of these issues to provide optimal, cost-effective care for patients.

Table 11.1 is a comprehensive list of gastroenterological medications and associated rheumatologic/musculoskeletal considerations. This chapter will focus on two major classes of medications: TNF inhibitors (TNF-Is) and proton pump inhibitors (PPIs).

Table 11.1 Musculoskeletal and Rheumatic Complications of Gastrointestinal Medications

Drugs	Rheumatic side effects
Antacids	Osteomalacia (aluminum hydroxide)
Surface agents/alginates (sucralfate)	Nil
H2 blockers	Polymyositis (cimetidine), arthralgia, myalgias, DRESS (famotidine)
PPI	Reduced BMD (via achlohydria), drug-induced lupus
Metoclopramide	Nil
Domperidone	Leg cramps
Macrolide abx	Azithro: photosensitivity, elevated CK
Cisapride	Nil
Pancreatic enzymes	Pancrealipase: muscle spasms, myalgia (post marketing)
Corticosteroids	Osteoporosis, myopathy, AVN

(Continued)

DOI: 10.1201/9781003367307-11

Table 11.1 (Continued) Musculoskeletal and Rheumatic Complications of Gastrointestinal Medications

Drugs	Rheumatic side effects
Rituximab	Serum sickness, lupus-like syndrome, arthralgia
Azathioprine	Azathioprine hypersensitivity
Ursodiol	Nil
Fenofibrates	DRESS, rhabdomylosis, photosensitivity
Calcineurin inhibitors: Cyclosporin, Tacro	Hyperuricaemia/gout (cyclosporin)
MTX	Nil
TNF inhibitors	Demyelinating disease, sarcoidosis-like drug reaction, drug-induced lupus, LCV, autoimmunity
Il-12/23 inhibitor: Stelara	Arthralgias (back)
Anti-integrin monoclonal antibody: Vedolizumab	Arthralgia
Jak-inhibitor: Tofacitinib	Arthralgias, MSK pain, tendinopathy
Sphingosine-1-phosphate receptor modulator (Ozanimod)	Arthralgias, back pain (< 3%)
Aminosalicylates: mesalamine, sulfsalazine	DRESS, EGPA, serum sickness, arthralgias (mesalamine) DRESS (SSZ)
Anti-alpha 4 integrin mab: Natalizumab	Arthralgia (8% to 19%), back (12%), limb pain (16%)
Il-23inhibitor: Skyrizi	Arthralgias (4–5% Crohn's)
Antidiarrhoeal: loperamide	Nil
Cholestyramine	Nil
Osmotic laxatives	Nil
Lubiprostone: chloride channel activator	Arthralgias, fibromyalgia syndrome
Guanylate cyclase agonists: Linaclotide, Plecanatide	Nil
Sodium/Hydrogen 3 (NHE 3) inhibitor: Tenapanor	Nil
Serotonin 4 receptor agonists: Tegaserod	< 2%: arthralgia, tendinopathy, elevated CK
Bile acid sequestrants	Nil
Serotonin 3 receptor antagonists: Alosetron	Muscle spasms, myalgias, skeletal pain
Eluxadoline	Nil
Rifaximin	Arthralgia, myalgia, muscle spasm, elevated CK
Dupilumab	Erythema nodosum, serum sickness, arthralgias and myalgias (3%), eosinophilia, EGPA
Fluoroquinolones	Arthralgias, tendon rupture
Tenofovir	Osteopenia, arthralgia, back pain
Entecavir	Nil
Direct-acting antivirals	Arthralgias, myalgias, asthenia, elevated CK (Sofosbuvir)
Midodrine	Asthenia, back pain, leg cramps
Octreotide	Arthralgia, asthenia
Terlipressin	Nil

Lexicomp. (n.d.). Drug information. *UpToDate*. Retrieved January 20, 2023 from www.uptodate.com/content

TNF INHIBITORS

TNF-alpha (TNFα) is a proinflammatory cytokine synthesized by activated macrophages and T cells. Binding of its receptors (TNFR1 [p55] and TNFR2 [p57]) stimulates release of other pro-inflammatory cytokines such as IL-1, IL-6, and IL-8, increases chemokine and endothelial adhesion molecule expression, and promotes leukocyte migration. Downstream effects include macrophage and phagocyte activation, monocyte differentiation, granuloma formation, and maintenance (1); these processes are integral to many disease states. Human and murine studies have shown the dichotomous effect of TNF (both reparatory and deleterious) in the various inflammatory stages leading to inflammatory bowel disease (IBD), whereas drugs blocking TNF help reduce IBD activity (2).

Since the late 1990s, TNF-Is have been used in the management of primary sclerosing cholangitis, microscopic colitis, and IBD. The FDA-approved TNF-Is for IBD are infliximab (chimeric human/murine 75%/25% IgG1 antibody), adalimumab, golimumab (fully human IgG1 antibodies), and certolizumab (pegylated Fab fragment of a humanized anti-TNF antibody) (3). Infliximab is an infusion, adalimumab and certolizumab are injectables, and golimumab is available in both formulations. Etanercept (human IgG1 Fc-tail TNF-receptor type 2 fusion protein) has not been shown to be effective for IBD.

RHEUMATOLOGIC CONSIDERATIONS

Immunogenicity

Immunogenicity describes the ability of a drug to induce an immunologic response and lead to the production of antibodies against itself (antidrug antibodies [ADAbs]). These can be nonneutralizing or neutralizing, resulting in decreased drug efficacy, worsened clinical disease, and increased likelihood of local and systemic adverse effects. ADAbs are a complication of TNF use (4, 5). Influencing factors include drug composition/structure, dosage, route of administration, and concomitant immunosuppressive comedication (3).

A systemic review of 68 studies (14,651 patients) examining the immunogenicity of TNF-Is in rheumatoid arthritis (RA), spondyloarthropathy (SpA), and IBD found the cumulative incidence of ADAbs was 12.7%. The individual incidence was 25.3% for infliximab, 14.1% adalimumab, 6.9% certolizumab, 3.8% golimumab, and 1.2% etanercept (4). A larger review of 443 studies found the highest overall rates with infliximab (0% to 83%), adalimumab (0% to 54%), and infliximab biosimilar CT-P13 (21% to 52%). Golimumab (0% to 19%) and etanercept (0% to 13%) had the lowest rates. Most ADAbs were neutralizing, except in the case of etanercept (6).

In a cohort of Crohn's patients with refractory luminal and fistulizing disease receiving Infliximab, ADAbs were detected in 61% by the fifth infusion, associated with infusion reactions and reduced treatment response (7). ADAbs formation was significantly associated with a loss of response and low drug trough levels in another combined IBD cohort (8). A comprehensive review of articles and abstracts between 2000 and 2012 in English and non-English literature revealed a higher risk of hypersensitivity reactions in patients with ADAbs regardless of underlying disease (RA, IBD, or SpA) (OR, 3.97; 95% CI, 2.36–6.67) (5).

Coadministration of immunosuppressive medications can reduce ADAbs formation and improve drug efficacy. Thomas et al. (4) found the odds of ADAbs were reduced by 74% with concomitant immunosuppressive use. In an earlier review (5), disease-modifying antirheumatic drugs, including azathioprine, decreased the risk of ADAbs seropositivity (OR 0.32; 95% CI, 0.25–0.42). Methotrexate 7.5 mg/week diminished the appearance of ADAbs in RA patients treated with 1, 3, and 10 mg/kg Infliximab (incidence rates of 15%, 7%, and 0%). The rates of ADAbs formation at the same doses without methotrexate were higher at 53%, 21%, and 7%, respectively (9). Baert (7) found that for Crohn's patients, there was a lower incidence of ADAbs with concomitant therapy (azathioprine, MTX, mesalamine, corticosteroids) than without (43% vs. 75%, $p < 0.01$). The use of AZA (2.25 mg/kg) or MTX (15 mg/week) lowered the incidence of ADAbs compared with infliximab monotherapy (46% vs. 73%; $p = 0.001$) in another Crohn's cohort of 174 patients. There was no significant difference between groups with respect to ADAbs development—MTX 44%, azathioprine 48% (10). Intravenous hydrocortisone pretreatment has been reported to reduce anti-infliximab antibody concentrations but not their formation (11).

Drug-Induced Lupus

Antinuclear (ANA) and double-stranded DNA (dsDNA) can be generated by TNF inhibitors. In prospective RA cohorts between 31% to 63% of infliximab-, 16% to 51% adalimumab-, and 12% to 48% of etanercept-treated patients had positive ANAs (12). Infliximab also induced ANAs in 52% of ankylosing spondylitis (AS), dsDNA ab in 9.5% of RA, and 2% AS (12). Reassuringly the overall incidence of DILE is, however, low, estimated between 0.5% and 1% (12), implying that detection of these autoantibodies should not be taken as evidence of impending disease.

Medications associated with drug-induced lupus erythematosus (DILE) can be stratified by their risk level and probability (definite, probable, or possible) of leading to the disease. There are four risk levels based on annual percentage incidence— high (> 5%), moderate (1–5%), low (0.1–1%), and very low (< 0.1%) (13, 14). Definite probability is based on reports from matched case-controlled studies, probable from cohort studies, and possible from case reports (13).

TNF-Is are classified as having a definite association but very low risk (12). However, with changes in prescription practices, this may shift. In a 2019 global pharmacovigilance study using the World Health Organization individual case safety report database (13), TNF-I were the most frequent drug family reported, accounting for 32.2% of cases. Among TNF cases, infliximab was the highest (12.2%), adalimumab 10.7%, and etanercept 8%. They were more commonly reported than procainamide and hydralazine, although the latter medications had the highest disproportionate reporting.

A 2003 French national survey estimated the frequency of lupus-like syndromes in patients treated with TNF inhibitors for rheumatic diseases to be comparable for infliximab (0.19%) and etanercept (0.18%) (15). Since then, most of the cases have been reported, with infliximab followed by etanercept and adalimumab (12, 16). Conversely, a 2014 disproportionality analysis study using a French pharmacovigilance database reported a higher odds ratio for adalimumab (ROR 9.03) than etanercept (ROR 4.02) (17).

The most common clinical manifestations of TNF-I-induced DILE are fever, inflammatory arthritis, and rash. The most common skin finding is subacute cutaneous lupus (annular and/or psoriasiform lesions) (Figure 11.1) occurring in sun-exposed areas and commonly in the upper back, neck, chest, and extensor surfaces of the arms (18).

Internal organ involvement such as lupus nephritis and serositis may occur, contrasting to that observed in classic DILE (16, 19). Positive DsDNA, extractable nuclear antigens, and low complements occur more frequently with TNF-induced disease than in the classic form, while anti-histone antibodies are less frequently reported (16).

Antiphospholipid antibody syndrome has also been described in patients treated with TNF blockers at an estimated incidence of 1% (20).

While exact mechanisms of pathogenesis have not been elucidated, several hypotheses exist. These include (15):

1. Release of antigenic material from cell apoptosis leading to autoantibody production and subsequent development of DIL
2. Disproportionate Th1 suppression in favor of Th2 causing production of interferons, which are important in the pathogenesis of lupus
3. Infections which are a consequence of TNF inhibition-inducing autoimmunity

Discontinuation of the offending medication is paramount to the management of DILE. The remaining manifestations are then treated based on the same strategies as for idiopathic disease. The prognosis is usually favorable, with resolution of symptoms, in most cases, within weeks to months.

Demyelinating Disease

Clinical trials with TNF-Is in multiple sclerosis (MS) were unfavorable and prematurely halted because of both clinical and radiographic disease exacerbations in TNF-I-treated patients (21). Their use has been associated with the development of MS, optic neuritis, acute transverse myelitis, Guillain–Barré and Miller Fisher syndromes, chronic inflammatory demyelinating polyneuropathy, multifocal motor neuropathy with conduction block, mononeuropathy multiplex, and axonal sensorimotor polyneuropathy (22). Representative demyelinating lesions on MRI are shown in Figure 11.2.

Demyelination occurs most frequently with infliximab (34% to 41% of reported cases), etanercept (30% to 47%), and adalimumab (19% to 23%). It is least frequent with certolizumab and golimumab (13, 23), but this may be because of lower prescription rates of these medications and their more recent emergence onto the market. This complication, however, remains uncommon. The raw incidence using the British RA registry data for TNF-I treated patients was estimated to be 19.7/100,000 patient-years with a standardized incidence rate of 1.38 (95% CI 0.96–1.92)

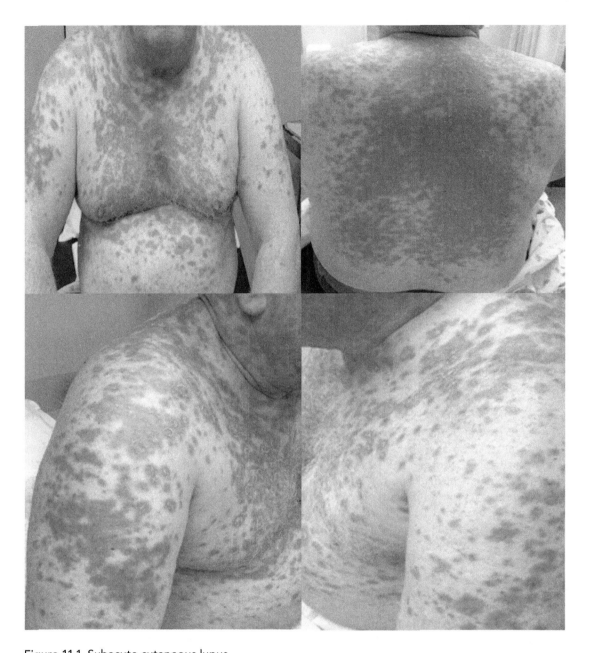

Figure 11.1 Subacute cutaneous lupus.

and 0.83 (0.51–1.26) limited to definite/probable cases (24).

TNF-Is are unable to cross the blood–brain barrier, and the precise pathogenesis to explain this complication is not fully understood. Possible mechanisms and theories have been advanced (11):

1. Permitting CNS ingress of peripheral autoreactive T cells

2. Downregulation of TNFR2 receptors needed for proliferation of oligodendrocytes and myelin repair

3. Changing cytokine milieu by increasing Il-12, interferon gamma and reducing Il-10, which creates a similar profile as for MS

4. Increasing TNFα in the CNS

5. Unmasking an underlying infection that could lead to autoimmune demyelination

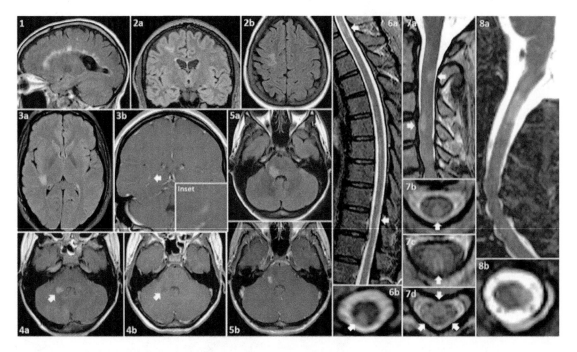

Figure 11.2 MRI images of TNF-I related CNS demyelination (reproduced with permission from Hutto SK, Rice DR, Mateen FJ. *J Neuroimmunol.* 2021;356:577587).

Symptoms of demyelination may include confusion, ataxia, dysesthesia, and paresthesia (25). Time to onset is variable after TNF-I initiation, ranging between 3 days and 12 years, with a mean of 17.61 months and median 3 years (11, 23).

A systematic review examining iatrogenic CNS demyelination identified 56 TNF-I-related cases between 2008 and 2018. All patients had TNF-Is discontinued. Thirty-three patients (58.9%) received steroids as treatment, and 9 patients received other therapeutics (intravenous immunoglobulin, plasma exchange, rituximab, and cyclophosphamide). The majority (78.5%) saw improvement in their condition, with 30.3% having complete resolution of neurological symptoms, leading to the conclusion that prognosis might be favorable upon medication discontinuation and steroid treatment (23). This, however, conflicts with the findings of a 2021 retrospective cohort study of 21 cases of TNF-I-induced CNS demyelination in which most patients suffered relapsing disease despite TNF-I discontinuation (26).

Psoriasis

Although utilized in the treatment of psoriasis and psoriatic arthritis, TNF-Is can lead to both de novo lesions and exacerbation of existing psoriasis. The pathogenesis is thought to be a result of the imbalance between TNFα- and type-1 interferons released from plasma dendritic cells (27).

A systematic review conducted between 1996 and 2009 found 207 cases of paradoxical psoriasis. Lesion morphology included pustular (56%), plaque (50%), guttate (12%), and mixed (15%). Fifty-nine percent of the cases were due to infliximab, 22% adalimumab, and 19% etanercept. The underlying diagnoses were RA (43%), SpA (26%), and IBD (20%) (28).

The prevalence of TNF-I-induced psoriasis in IBD is estimated at 1.6% to 2.7% (29), with an incidence of 6.9% for psoriasiform lesions and 4.6% for psoriasis based on data from a systematic review and meta-analysis of 24,547 IBD patients (30). In this review, a statistically higher risk was observed in female patients (OR 1.46), those who were younger at TNF-I (OR 1.03), smokers (OR 1.97), those with ileocolonic Crohn's disease (OR 1.48), and use of adalimumab or certolizumab (OR: 1.48 and 2.87, respectively vs. infliximab) (30).

Comparatively, the prevalence of TNF-I-induced psoriasis in RA patients is approximately 2.3% to 5% (29). Adalimumab treated individuals have a significantly higher incident rate compared with etanercept (IRR 4.6) and infliximab (IRR 3.5) (31).

Sarcoidosis

A 2009 French observational study described 10 patients with RA and spondyloarthritis who developed biopsy-proven sarcoidosis-like granulomatosis following TNF-I initiation. This study estimated the incidence to be very low (1:2800 [0.04%]) (32).

In a 2017 review of 90 reported cases, etanercept was most frequently implicated (n = 53, 59%), nearly thrice that for adalimumab (n = 21, 23%) and infliximab (n = 16, 18%). The median age was 43 years, with a female predominance. RA was the predominant underlying disease, followed by AS and psoriasiform arthritis; IBD accounted for six cases. In 71 cases, there was at least a partial resolution by stopping treatment, initiation of steroids, or both. Re-initiation of TNF-Is caused relapse in 7 out of 20 cases. Median duration between therapy initiation and diagnosis was 22.5 months (range 1–84 months), with lungs (n = 67, including hilar and mediastinal lymphadenopathy), skin (n = 31), and eyes (n = 12) affected most (33).

Vasculitis

Between January 1990 and December 2006, 113 cases of drug-induced vasculitis were reported (34), occurring at a mean of 38 weeks on therapy (etanercept 59, infliximab 47, adalimumab 5, and other agents 2). It was biopsy proven in 73%: leukocytoclastic in 52 patients (63%), necrotizing in 14 (17%), and lymphocytic in 5 (6%). Ninety-eight patients (87%) had skin involvement such as purpura, cutaneous ulcers, nodules, digital vasculitis, or maculopapular rash. Twenty-seven patients (24%) had internal involvement manifesting with peripheral neuropathy (16%), renal (13%), CNS (4%), and pulmonary (3%) disease. Gallbladder, temporal arterial, and cardiac involvement accounted for one case each. ANA was positive in 27 cases, ANCA in 10, cryoglobulins in 5, DsDNA in 4, antiphospholipid antibodies in 3, SSA/B in 1.

Of the outcome detailed in 100 cases, 67 completely resolved, 25 partially and 8 without resolution.

Interstitial Lung Disease

Between January 1990 and December 2006, 24 cases of TNF-I-associated interstitial lung disease (ILD) were described. Disorders included interstitial pneumonitis (n = 18), sarcoidosis (n = 3), pulmonary hemorrhage (n = 2), and bronchiolitis obliterans organizing pneumonia (n = 1). Infliximab accounted for 19 cases (79%), etanercept 4 (17%), and adalimumab 1 (4%). ILD appeared after a mean of 42 weeks of treatment. Despite therapy cessation, prognosis was poor. Resolution was observed in only 9 patients (47%), with permanent disease in 10 (53%). Six patients subsequently died (32%), but four of these had a previous diagnosis of ILD (34). It is worth noting that while ILD has been described in IBD as an association (35–37), this remains both rare and poorly defined, confounded by other variables, and may in fact be more likely due to drug effects.

Autoimmune Hepatitis

One report described seven cases of Infliximab-induced autoimmune hepatitis between 1990 and 2008 (38). In 2015, Rodriguez et al. documented a further eight cases (seven infliximab) based on biopsies with consistent features of chronic lymphoplasmocytic infiltrate and interface hepatitis. Treatment with steroids was effective, and only two patients required long-term therapy (39). Case reports also exist implicating adalimumab as the inciting agent (40–43).

Myositis

There have been approximately 25 documented cases of TNF-I-associated myositis: 18 in inflammatory arthritis (16 RA, 1 JIA, 2 AS) and 2 cases with IBD (1 CD, 1 UC). The triggering drugs were evenly divided across the class, with etanercept in eight patients, followed by infliximab (seven), adalimumab (four), three combined (two on ETN/ADA; one ADA/IFX), Lenercept (two) (44).

PROTON PUMP INHIBITORS

Background

PPIs reduce gastric acid secretion by irreversibly binding to the hydrogen-potassium-ATPase pump of the parietal cell membrane. They are used in the treatment of GERD, Barrett's esophagus, and hypersecretory conditions and as prophylaxis of peptic ulcer disease (45). Since omeprazole's introduction in 1989, there are now an additional five FDA-approved PPIs: esomeprazole, lansoprazole, pantoprazole, dexlansoprazole, and rabendazole (6). The latter two medications are only available as oral formulations.

Recently, there has been a concern that PPIs may increase autoimmune diseases, possibly by altering the host intestinal microbiome. A 2021 retrospective cohort population-based study (46) of 298,000 patients found a higher rate of both organ-specific and systemic autoimmune diseases in patients taking PPIs regardless of dose. Elevated risks of celiac disease (47) and inflammatory bowel disease (48) have also been observed. While there has been a case report of omeprazole-induced dermatomyositis (49), a later case-control study did not support an association between PPIs and inflammatory myopathies (50). These observed associations may be confounded by the high frequency of PPI prescriptions in patients with connective tissue diseases in whom GERD is a frequent finding.

RHEUMATOLOGIC CONSIDERATIONS

Drug-Induced Cutaneous Lupus Erythematosus

In a Swedish case-control study, 66 out of 234 DICLE cases between 2006 and 2009 were found to be associated with PPI (OR 2.9) (51). In a retrospective study in the English literature between 8/2009 and 6/2016, PPIs accounted for the greatest number of reported cases, with the incidence increasing by 34.1% (52) whereas the incidence for biologics was 11.4%. Of 448 confirmed cases of cutaneous lupus diagnosed at Danish University Hospital between 1994 and 2014, 88 cases were drug-induced, and the greatest portion (> 25%) was due to PPIs (53).

A matched case-control study between 2009 and 2019 sought to compare primary SCLE to PPI-induced SCLE. Omeprazole accounted for the highest number (25), then lansoprazole (9), pantoprazole (1), and esomeprazole (1). Figure 11.3 shows one patient from the study. One of the most significant findings was the distribution of lesions in PPI-induced SCLE, with 72% of patients having lower limb involvement compared to 7% of patients with

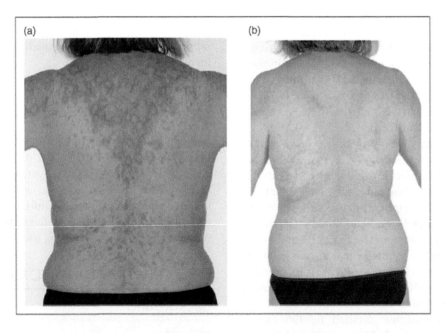

Figure 11.3 A picture showing (a) Omeprazole-induced SCLE and (b) after Omeprazole discontinuation. Reproduced with permission from Poh YJ, Alrashid A, Sangle SR et al. *Lupus*. 2022;31(9):1078–83.

primary disease ($p < 0.0001$). Lesions of the sun-exposed areas of the trunk, face, and upper extremities were similar in both groups. Anti-Ro-52 antibodies were numerically higher in the PPI group (60% vs. 42% primary group). Anti-Smith and Anti-dsDNA were similar in both (Smith—18% PPI, 23% primary; DsDNA—36% PPI, 38% primary). The authors concluded that lower limb involvement is an indicator of PPI-induced SCLE (18). To date, there have been no reported cases of PPI-induced systemic lupus erythematosus.

Metabolic Bone Effects

In 2010, the FDA issued a warning about the potential for increased risk of spine, wrist, and hip fractures with chronic use (54).

Prospective data has demonstrated PPI use to be associated with:

1. A shorter time to first nontraumatic fracture (HR 1.75)—a persistent relationship after controlling for multiple risk factors including femoral neck bone density (HR 1.40) (55).
2. An increased risk of subsequent osteoporosis medication use (Sub Hazard Ratio 1.28) and fractures (SHR 1.29) when compared to PPI nonuse. The risk of fracture was greatest with rabeprazole (SHR 2.06) (56).

A case-control study of 10,958 patients in the United Kingdom revealed a moderately increased risk of hip fractures (OR 1.09), more so with medium (OR 1.11) and high doses (1.31) unrelated to length of use (57).

A meta-analysis of 18 observational studies demonstrated that PPIs increased the risk of spine fractures, hip fractures, and fractures at any site by 58%, 26%, and 33%, respectively, regardless of the duration of use (58).

There was a 39% increase in odds of fracture amongst young adults (18–29 years) OR 1.39 (95% CI 1.26–1.53), while the increase in children (4–17) was not statistically significant OR 1.13 (95% CI 0.92–1.39). The most common fracture sites were wrist (24.9%) and hand (20.5%) in children, foot (12.4%) and hand (32.5%) for young adults (59).

The overall hip fracture risk was higher in men above 45 years who had used omeprazole and pantoprazole in a case-control study of 6,774 matched pairs (OR 1.13, 95% CI 1.01–1.27).

The exact mechanism of fracture risk has not been elucidated. Hypotheses include elevation in parathyroid hormone levels (due to an increase in parathyroid gene expression, hyperplasia, and hypertrophy of the parathyroid glands) as a downstream effect of hypergastrinaemia; the hypochlorhydric effect on micronutrient absorption leading to hypocalcaemia, hypomagnesaemia and low B12 (60); impairment of osteoblastic activity (61, 62), and a possible increase in osteoclastic activity (63).

While fracture risk is increased, there is no clear evidence that PPI use directly leads to osteoporosis. This was demonstrated in a study prospectively assessing the relationship between PPI use and bone mineral density (BMD) of the lumbar spine (vertebrae L1-L4), femoral neck, and total hip. BMD was assessed at baseline then after 5 and 10 years of PPI use. At baseline, 8,340 subjects were included, and PPI use was associated with a significantly lower BMD at both the femoral neck and total hip. However, at the 5- and 10-year follow-up, accelerated BMD loss was not observed in PPI users (64).

Currently, routine BMD screening is not recommended for patients on long-term PPIs.

Effect on Mycophenolate Absorption

Mycophenolate mofetil (MMF) is used to manage end organ manifestations in several rheumatic diseases. Patients with these diseases frequently have co-morbid GERD and are on PPIs.

MMF exacts its immunosuppressive effect by impairing B and T cell function through reversible inhibition of inosine monophosphate dehydrogenase. The acidic gastric environment is responsible for converting MMF to the active metabolite (MPA). Coadministration of pantoprazole was shown to significantly reduce the maximum peak concentrations of MMF by 60% in a small trial of 36 patients with stable autoimmune disease (65) and lowered MPA plasma concentrations in cardiac transplant recipients (66). However, in a study of renal transplant patients, pantoprazole had no impact on the immunosuppressive effect of MPA despite influencing the pharmacokinetics of MMF (67).

It is not feasible for PPIs to be withheld completely in many patients with connective tissue diseases. While no formal guidelines exist, it has been suggested that MMF drug levels be monitored in order to avoid therapeutic failure (68) and that administration times be staggered to allow maximal MMF absorption.

VEDOLIZUMAB

Vedolizumab is a humanized monoclonal antibody that ultimately prevents T cell migration into intestinal mucosal layers by binding to alpha4beta7 integrin, thus preventing its interaction with mucosal addressing cell adhesion molecule-1. The Varsity trial (69) found vedolizumab to be superior to adalimumab for moderate to severe ulcerative colitis and presented it as an increasingly popular choice to gastroenterologists. It is FDA approved for IBD.

Data regarding its effects on articular manifestations of IBD is conflicting. No efficacy was reported in a retrospective observational study of 171 treated patients (70), while a smaller case series showed active spondyloarthritis symptoms began soon after therapy was started (71, 72). Conversely, a prospective observational study showed a benefit (73). When compared to ustekinumab, vedoluzimab-related arthralgias were transient, and in fact, worsening of pre-existing arthralgia was the same for both medications (74). A 2022 meta-analysis of 2466 patients reported 13% of vedolizumab patients and 10% of placebo patients developed arthralgias/arthritis of any kind, without statistical significance. The authors concluded that new-onset or worsening articular symptoms are due to the course of disease itself, the body's response to drugs, or exclusion of steroids from treatment (75).

DRUG HYPERSENSITIVITY

Drug Reaction with Eosinophilia and Systemic Symptoms

The aminosalicylates, which include sulfasalazine and mesalamine, are used as a first-line therapy for the management and remission maintenance of mild to moderate ulcerative colitis (76). The efficacy in Crohn's disease, however, is less certain (77, 78).

Sulfasalazine is reported to be the second most common cause of drug reaction with eosinophilia and systemic symptoms (DRESS) after allopurinol, amongst drugs used in the treatment of rheumatic diseases (79).

DRESS or drug-induced hypersensitivity (DIH) reaction is a delayed T cell–mediated process comprising severe cutaneous eruptions associated with fever, lymphadenopathy, hematologic abnormalities, multisystem involvement, and viral reactivation (human herpes virus 6, Epstein Barr virus, and cytomegalovirus) (80). It usually begins 2 weeks to 2 months after drug initiation (81). The different diagnostic criteria for this syndrome are presented in Figure 11.4.

The cutaneous manifestations (Figure 11.5) are varied and may consist of maculopapular/

Table 1 Comparison of criteria for the diagnosis of DRESS/DIHS

Bocquet et al.[6]	Japanese Consensus Group[7]	RegiSCAR[12]
1. A cutaneous drug eruption 2. Systemic involvement lymphadenopathy ≥ 2 cm in diameter or hepatitis (transaminase ≥ 2 times upper limit of normal) or interstitial nephritis or interstitial pneumonitis or carditis 3. Hematologic abnormalities eosinophilia $\geq 1.5 \times 10^9/L$ or presence of atypical lymphocytes	1. Maculopapular eruption developing >3 weeks after starting a limited number of drugs 2. Prolonged clinical manifestations 2 weeks after discontinuation of the causative drug 3. Fever (>38°C) 4. Liver abnormalities (alanine aminotransferase >100 U/L) * 5. Leukocyte abnormalities (at least 1 present): • Leukocytosis (>11 × 10⁹/L) • Atypical lymphocytosis (>5%) • Eosinophilia (>1.5 × 10⁹/L) 6. Lymphadenopathy 7. HHV-6 reactivation	1. Acute skin eruption 2. Fever (>38°C) 3. Lymphadenopathy at ≥ 2 sites 4. Involvement of at least 1 internal organ 5. Lymphocytosis or lymphocytopenia 6. Peripheral eosinophilia 7. Thrombocytopenia
The presence of all 3 is required.	The diagnosis is confirmed by the presence of all criteria (typical DIHS) or the first 5 (atypical DIHS).	The presence of at least 3 of the characteristics is required for the diagnosis of DRESS. In addition, a scoring system[12] is applied to classify patients as *definite*, *probably*, or *no case*.

DIHS, drug-induced hypersensitivity reaction; DRESS, drug reaction with eosinophilia and systemic clinical manifestations; HHV, human herpes virus.
    * This can be replaced by other organ involvement, such as renal involvement.

Figure 11.4 DRESS diagnostic criteria comparison table. Reproduced with permission (80).

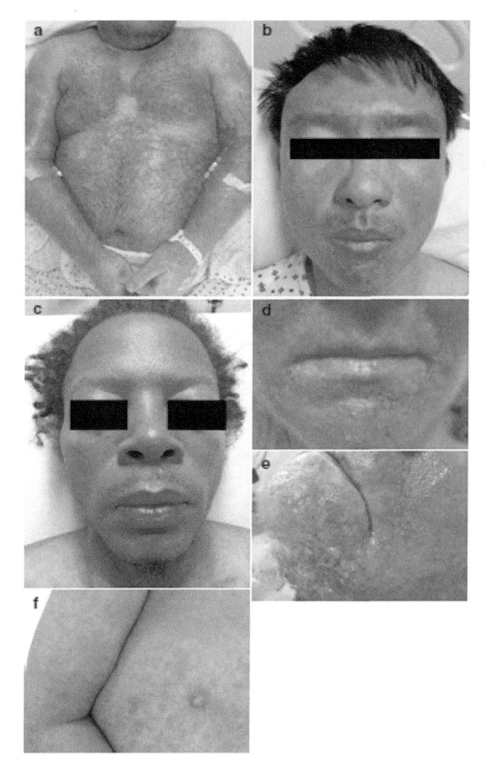

Figure 11.5 The variety of cutaneous findings in DRESS syndrome. Reproduced with permission from Chang, A.Y. (2018). Drug Rash with Eosinophilia and Systemic Symptoms. In: Rosenbach, M., Wanat, K., Micheletti, R., Taylor, L. (eds) *Inpatient Dermatology*. Springer, Cham.

morbilliform lesions, erythroderma, toxic epidermal necrolysis, Stevens-Johnson syndrome, erythema multiforme, or a purpuric rash (79).

The most common histopathologic pattern of DIH/DRESS is spongiotic dermatitis with eosinophils with a perivascular lymphocytic infiltrate in the dermis (81). In reports of Sulfasalazine-induced DRESS, the liver was the most commonly involved organ (approximately 72% of cases), followed by the kidney (79).

The prognosis is variable. Disease activity can continue after discontinuation of the offending drug, and relapses can occur in up to 25% of patients (80). The mortality rate is approximately 10% (82).

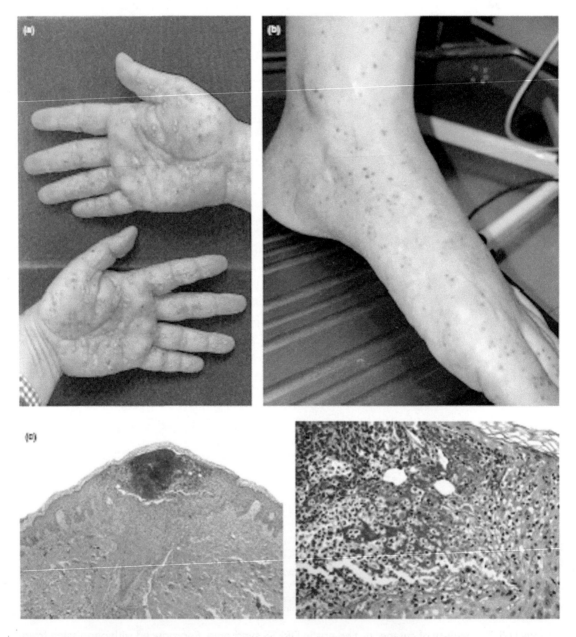

Figure 11.6 Azathioprine hypersensitivity. This figure shows (a) papulosquamous lesions on both hands; (b) lower extremity petechiae; (c) histopathology of a pustule with perivascular and interstitial inflammatory infiltrates rich in neutrophils (x20); (d) higher magnification of the neutrophil aggregates (x200). Reproduced with permission (83).

Short-term complications (within weeks after onset) include myocarditis, fulminant hepatic failure, pneumonitis, and gastrointestinal bleeding (84).

Autoimmune sequelae including SLE (85, 86), autoimmune thyroiditis, vitiligo, myocarditis, and rheumatoid arthritis (81) have been described as long-term complications of DRESS, appearing months up to as long as 9 years after resolution of skin eruptions and acute systemic involvement (81, 86).

In a retrospective cohort of 55 DRESS patients followed longitudinally for 18 years, nine progressed to autoimmune sequelae regardless of treatment. The generation of autoantibodies was preceded by 8 years. Increases in lymphocyte counts, severe liver damage, rebound increase in globulin, persistent reactivation of EBV and HHV-6, low IL-2 and IL-4 at the acute phases were identified as risk factors for future development of autoimmune disease. A scoring system has been proposed to identify high-risk patients (86).

Systemic corticosteroids are the mainstay of treatment in doses between 0.5 and 1 mg/kg/day (84). To prevent relapse of various symptoms, they are tapered over 6 to 12 weeks (84) or up to a year in protracted cases. Refractory cases may warrant the use of immunosuppressive therapy, and reports exist of successful treatment with cyclosporine, mycophenolate, rituximab, plasmapheresis, cyclophosphamide, and IVIG 0.5–1 mg/kg/day over 2 days (81).

Azathioprine Hypersensitivity

Azathioprine hypersensitivity is an idiosyncratic non–IgE-mediated allergic reaction, occurring within the first 4 weeks of therapy, independent of TPMT levels (87). It is rare, experienced by 2% of patients initiating therapy (88). Between 1986 and 2009, Bindinger et al. (89) found 67 cases reported in the English literature, 49% of which had an underlying diagnosis of either inflammatory bowel disease or multiple sclerosis. This led them to suggest that patients with these diagnoses were at increased risk of developing the syndrome.

The clinical features vary but may consist of fever, malaise, arthralgia/myalgia, vomiting, diarrhea, or rash. Leukocytosis and abnormal liver function are frequent laboratory findings. Occasionally, renal dysfunction, hypotension, and shock may be present (89), in some cases severe enough to mimic sepsis (90).

The skin findings (Figure 11.6), which may be present in approximately 50% of patients, have included maculopapular, vesicular, pustular, purpuric, urticarial, and erythema nodosum eruptions. Histopathologically, a neutrophilic dermatosis predominates (88) but leukocytoclastic vasculitis has also been observed (90).

If appropriately recognized, the prognosis is favorable, with improvement on drug cessation. Continuation or rechallenge can have potentially life-threatening complications and is thus contraindicated (88).

CONCLUSION

Medications for gastrointestinal diseases can have a myriad of rheumatic implications. As these medications are prescribed more widely, knowledge of these complications should assist in early recognition and timely intervention to prevent morbidity and mortality in the patients for whom they are prescribed.

REFERENCES

1. Koo S, Marty FM, Baden LR. Infectious complications associated with immunomodulating biologic agents. *Infect Dis Clin North Am*. 2010;24(2):285–306.
2. Pagnini C, Cominelli F. Tumor necrosis factor's pathway in Crohn's disease: Potential for intervention. *Int J Mol Sci*. 2021;22(19):10273.
3. Atiqi S, Hooijberg F, Loeff FC et al. Immunogenicity of TNF-inhibitors. *Front Immunol*. 2020;11:312.
4. Thomas SS, Borazan N, Barroso N et al. Comparative immunogenicity of TNF inhibitors: Impact on clinical efficacy and tolerability in the management of autoimmune diseases: A systematic review and meta-analysis. *BioDrugs*. 2015;29(4):241–58.
5. Maneiro JR, Salgado E, Gomez-Reino JJ. Immunogenicity of monoclonal antibodies against tumor necrosis factor used in chronic immune-mediated Inflammatory conditions: Systematic review and meta-analysis. *JAMA Intern Med*. 2013;173(15):1416–28.
6. Strand DS, Kim D, Peura DA. 25 years of proton pump inhibitors: A comprehensive review. *Gut Liver*. 2017;11(1):27–37.

7. Baert F, Noman M, Vermeire S et al. Influence of immunogenicity on the long-term efficacy of infliximab in Crohn's disease. *N Engl J Med.* 2003;348(7):601–8.

8. Steenholdt C, Bendtzen K, Brynskov J et al. Cut-off levels and diagnostic accuracy of infliximab trough levels and anti-infliximab antibodies in Crohn's disease. *Scand J Gastroenterol.* 2011;46(3):310–8.

9. Maini RN, Breedveld FC, Kalden JR et al. Therapeutic efficacy of multiple intravenous infusions of anti-tumor necrosis factor alpha monoclonal antibody combined with low-dose weekly methotrexate in rheumatoid arthritis. *Arthritis Rheum.* 1998;41(9):1552–63.

10. Vermeire S, Noman M, Van Assche G et al. Effectiveness of concomitant immunosuppressive therapy in suppressing the formation of antibodies to infliximab in Crohn's disease. *Gut.* 2007;56(9):1226–31.

11. Farrell RJ, Alsahli M, Jeen YT et al. Intravenous hydrocortisone premedication reduces antibodies to infliximab in Crohn's disease: A randomized controlled trial. *Gastroenterol.* 2003;124(4):917–24.

12. Araujo-Fernandez S, Ahijon-Lana M, Isenberg DA. Drug-induced lupus: Including anti-tumour necrosis factor and interferon induced. *Lupus.* 2014;23(6):545–53.

13. Vaglio A, Grayson PC, Fenaroli P et al. Drug-induced lupus: Traditional and new concepts. *Autoimmun Rev.* 2018;17(9):912–18.

14. Arnaud L, Mertz P, Gavand PE et al. Drug-induced systemic lupus: Revisiting the ever-changing spectrum of the disease using the WHO pharmacovigilance database. *Ann Rheum Dis.* 2019;78(4):504–8.

15. De Bandt M, Sibilia J, Le Loet X et al. Systemic lupus erythematosus induced by anti-tumour necrosis factor alpha therapy: A French national survey. *Arthritis Res Ther.* 2005;7(3):R545–51.

16. Skalkou A, Pelechas E, Voulgari PV et al. TNF-induced Lupus: A case-based review. *Curr Rheumatol Rev.* 2022;18(1):72–82.

17. Moulis G, Sommet A, Lapeyre-Mestre M et al. Association Francaise des centres regionaux de P: Is the risk of tumour necrosis factor inhibitor-induced lupus or lupus-like syndrome the same with monoclonal antibodies and soluble receptor? A case/non-case study in a nationwide pharmacovigilance database. *Rheumatol (Oxford).* 2014;53(10):1864–71.

18. Poh YJ, Alrashid A, Sangle SR et al. Proton pump inhibitor induced subacute cutaneous lupus erythematosus: Clinical characteristics and outcomes. *Lupus.* 2022;31(9):1078–83.

19. Costa MF, Said NR, Zimmermann B. Drug-induced lupus due to anti-tumor necrosis factor alpha agents. *Semin Arthritis Rheum.* 2008;37(6):381–7.

20. Boyman O, Comte D, Spertini F. Adverse reactions to biologic agents and their medical management. *Nat Rev Rheumatol.* 2014;10(10):612–27.

21. Kemanetzoglou E, Andreadou E. CNS demyelination with TNF-alpha blockers. *Curr Neurol Neurosci Rep.* 2017;17(4):36.

22. Baker D, Hadjicharalambous C, Gnanapavan S et al. Can rheumatologists stop causing demyelinating disease? *Mult Scler Relat Disord.* 2021;53:103057.

23. Kumar N, Abboud H. Iatrogenic CNS demyelination in the era of modern biologics. *Mult Scler.* 2019;25(8):1079–85.

24. Taylor TRP, Galloway J, Davies R et al. Demyelinating events following initiation of anti-TNFalpha therapy in the British society for rheumatology biologics registry in rheumatoid arthritis. *Neurol Neuroimmunol Neuroinflamm.* 2021;8(3).

25. Mohan N, Edwards ET, Cupps TR et al. Demyelination occurring during anti-tumor necrosis factor alpha therapy for inflammatory arthritides. *Arthritis Rheum.* 2001;44(12):2862–9.

26. Hutto SK, Rice DR, Mateen FJ. CNS demyelination with TNFalpha inhibitor exposure: A retrospective cohort study. *J Neuroimmunol.* 2021;356:577587.

27. Mylonas A, Conrad C. Psoriasis: Classical vs. paradoxical: The Yin-Yang of TNF and Type I interferon. *Front Immunol.* 2018;9:2746.

28. Collamer AN, Battafarano DF. Psoriatic skin lesions induced by tumor necrosis factor antagonist therapy: Clinical features and possible immunopathogenesis. *Semin Arthritis Rheum.* 2010;40(3):233–40.

29. Li SJ, Perez-Chada LM, Merola JF. TNF inhibitor-induced psoriasis: Proposed algorithm for treatment and management. *J Psoriasis Psoriatic Arthritis.* 2019;4(2):70–80.

30. Xie W, Xiao S, Huang H et al. Incidence of and risk factors for paradoxical psoriasis or psoriasiform lesions in inflammatory bowel disease patients receiving anti-TNF therapy: Systematic review with meta-analysis. *Front Immunol.* 2022;13:847160.

31. Harrison MJ, Dixon WG, Watson KD et al. Rates of new-onset psoriasis in patients with rheumatoid arthritis receiving anti-tumour necrosis factor alpha therapy: Results from the British society for rheumatology biologics register. *Ann Rheum Dis.* 2009;68(2):209–15.

32. Daien CI, Monnier A, Claudepierre P et al. Sarcoid-like granulomatosis in patients treated with tumor necrosis factor blockers: 10 cases. *Rheumatol* (Oxford). 2009;48(8):883–6.

33. Decock A, Van Assche G, Vermeire S et al. Sarcoidosis-like lesions: Another paradoxical reaction to anti-TNF therapy? *J Crohns Colitis.* 2017;11(3):378–83.

34. Ramos-Casals M, Brito-Zeron P, Munoz S et al. Autoimmune diseases induced by TNF-targeted therapies: Analysis of 233 cases. *Med* (Baltimore). 2007;86(4):242–51.

35. Hoffmann RM, Kruis W. Rare extraintestinal manifestations of inflammatory bowel disease. *Inflamm Bowel Dis.* 2004;10(2):140–7.

36. Betancourt SL, Palacio D, Jimenez CA et al. Thoracic manifestations of inflammatory bowel disease. *AJR Am J Roentgenol.* 2011;197(3):W452–6.

37. Ji XQ, Wang LX, Lu DG. Pulmonary manifestations of inflammatory bowel disease. *World J Gastroenterol.* 2014;20(37):13501–11.

38. Ramos-Casals M, Brito-Zeron P, Soto MJ et al. Autoimmune diseases induced by TNF-targeted therapies. *Best Pract Res Clin Rheumatol.* 2008;22(5):847–61.

39. Rodrigues S, Lopes S, Magro F et al. Autoimmune hepatitis and anti-tumor necrosis factor alpha therapy: A single center report of 8 cases. *World J Gastroenterol.* 2015;21(24):7584–8.

40. Adar T, Mizrahi M, Pappo O et al. Adalimumab-induced autoimmune hepatitis. *J Clin Gastroenterol.* 2010;44(1):e20–2.

41. Grasland A, Sterpu R, Boussoukaya S et al. Autoimmune hepatitis induced by adalimumab with successful switch to abatacept. *Eur J Clin Pharmacol.* 2012;68(5):895–8.

42. Borman MA, Urbanski S, Swain MG. Anti-TNF-induced autoimmune hepatitis. *J Hepatol.* 2014;61(1):169–70.

43. Miranda-Bautista J, Menchen L. Adalimumab-induced autoimmune hepatitis in a patient with Crohn's disease. *Gastroenterol Hepatol.* 2019;42(5):306–7.

44. Yoshida A, Katsumata Y, Hirahara S et al. Tumour necrosis factor inhibitor-induced myositis in a patient with ulcerative colitis. *Mod Rheumatol Case Rep.* 2021;5(1):156–61.

45. Freedberg DE, Kim LS, Yang YX. The risks and benefits of long-term use of proton pump inhibitors: Expert review and best practice advice from the American gastroenterological association. *Gastroenterol.* 2017;152(4):706–15.

46. Lin SH, Chang YS, Lin TM et al. Proton pump inhibitors increase the risk of autoimmune diseases: A nationwide cohort study. *Front Immunol.* 2021;12:736036.

47. Lebwohl B, Spechler SJ, Wang TC et al. Use of proton pump inhibitors and subsequent risk of celiac disease. *Dig Liver Dis.* 2014;46(1):36–40.

48. Xia B, Yang M, Nguyen LH et al. Regular use of proton pump inhibitor and the risk of inflammatory bowel disease: Pooled analysis of 3 prospective cohorts. *Gastroenterol.* 2021;161(6):1842–52 e10.

49. Pan Y, Chong AH, Williams RA et al. Omeprazole-induced dermatomyositis. *Br J Dermatol.* 2006;154(3):557–8.

50. Khoo T, Caughey GE, Hill C et al. Proton pump inhibitors are not associated with inflammatory myopathies: A case control study. *Muscle Nerve.* 2018;58(6):855–7.

51. Gronhagen CM, Fored CM, Linder M et al. Subacute cutaneous lupus erythematosus and its association with drugs: A population-based matched case-control study of 234 patients in Sweden. *Br J Dermatol.* 2012;167(2):296–305.

52. Michaelis TC, Sontheimer RD, Lowe GC. An update in drug-induced subacute cutaneous lupus erythematosus. *Dermatol Online J*. 2017;23(3).

53. Laurinaviciene R, Sandholdt LH, Bygum A. Drug-induced cutaneous lupus erythematosus: 88 new cases. *Eur J Dermatol*. 2017;27(1):28–33.

54. Chinzon D, Domingues G, Tosetto N et al. Safety of long-term proton pump inhibitors: Facts and myths. *Arq Gastroenterol*. 2022;59(2):219–25.

55. Fraser LA, Leslie WD, Targownik LE et al. The effect of proton pump inhibitors on fracture risk: Report from the Canadian Multicenter Osteoporosis Study. *Osteoporos Int*. 2013;24(4):1161–8.

56. van der Hoorn MMC, Tett SE, de Vries OJ et al. The effect of dose and type of proton pump inhibitor use on risk of fractures and osteoporosis treatment in older Australian women: A prospective cohort study. *Bone*. 2015;81:675–82.

57. Cea Soriano L, Ruigomez A, Johansson S et al. Study of the association between hip fracture and acid-suppressive drug use in a UK primary care setting. *Pharmacotherapy*. 2014;34(6):570–81.

58. Zhou B, Huang Y, Li H et al. Proton-pump inhibitors and risk of fractures: An update meta-analysis. *Osteoporos Int*. 2016;27(1):339–47.

59. Freedberg DE, Haynes K, Denburg MR et al. Use of proton pump inhibitors is associated with fractures in young adults: A population-based study. *Osteoporos Int*. 2015;26(10):2501–7.

60. Thong BKS, Ima-Nirwana S, Chin KY. Proton pump inhibitors and fracture risk: A review of current evidence and mechanisms involved. *Int J Environ Res Public Health*. 2019;16(9).

61. Cheng Z, Liu Y, Ma M et al. Lansoprazole-induced osteoporosis via the IP3R- and SOCE-mediated calcium signaling pathways. *Mol Med*. 2022;28(1):21.

62. Desai BV, Qadri MN, Vyas BA. Proton pump inhibitors and osteoporosis risk: Exploring the role of TRPM7 channel. *Eur J Clin Pharmacol*. 2022;78(1):35–41.

63. Jo Y, Park E, Ahn SB et al. A proton pump inhibitor's effect on bone metabolism mediated by osteoclast action in old age: A prospective randomized study. *Gut Liver*. 2015;9(5):607–14.

64. Targownik LE, Leslie WD, Davison KS et al. The relationship between proton pump inhibitor use and longitudinal change in bone mineral density: A population-based study [corrected] from the Canadian Multicentre Osteoporosis Study (CaMos). *Am J Gastroenterol*. 2012;107(9):1361–9.

65. Schaier M, Scholl C, Scharpf D et al. Proton pump inhibitors interfere with the immunosuppressive potency of mycophenolate mofetil. *Rheumatol* (Oxford). 2010;49(11):2061–7.

66. Kofler S, Deutsch MA, Bigdeli AK et al. Proton pump inhibitor co-medication reduces mycophenolate acid drug exposure in heart transplant recipients. *J Heart Lung Transplant*. 2009;28(6):605–11.

67. Rissling O, Glander P, Hambach P et al. No relevant pharmacokinetic interaction between pantoprazole and mycophenolate in renal transplant patients: A randomized crossover study. *Br J Clin Pharmacol*. 2015;80(5):1086–96.

68. Alex G, Shanoj KC, Reachel Varghese D et al. Co-prescription of anti-acid therapy reduces the bioavailability of mycophenolate mofetil in systemic sclerosis patients. *Ann Rheum Dis*. 2021;80(Suppl 1):700–1.

69. Sands BE, Peyrin-Biroulet L, Loftus EV, Jr. et al. Vedolizumab versus adalimumab for moderate-to-severe ulcerative colitis. *N Engl J Med*. 2019;381(13):1215–26.

70. Paccou J, Nachury M, Duchemin C et al. Vedolizumab has no efficacy on articular manifestations in patients with spondyloarthritis associated with inflammatory bowel disease. *Joint Bone Spine*. 2019;86(5):654–6.

71. Varkas G, Thevissen K, De Brabanter G et al. An induction or flare of arthritis and/or sacroiliitis by vedolizumab in inflammatory bowel disease: A case series. *Ann Rheum Dis*. 2017;76(5):878–81.

72. Dubash S, Marianayagam T, Tinazzi I et al. Emergence of severe spondyloarthr

opathy-related entheseal pathology following successful vedolizumab therapy for inflammatory bowel disease. *Rheumatol (Oxford).* 2019;58(6):963–8.

73. Orlando A, Orlando R, Ciccia F et al. Clinical benefit of vedolizumab on articular manifestations in patients with active spondyloarthritis associated with inflammatory bowel disease. *Ann Rheum Dis.* 2017;76(9):e31.

74. De Galan C, Truyens M, Peeters H et al. The impact of Vedolizumab and Ustekinumab on articular extra-intestinal manifestations in inflammatory bowel disease patients: A real-life multicentre cohort study. *J Crohns Colitis.* 2022;16(11):1676–86.

75. dos Anjos GA, Gomes CP, Oliveira DB et al. Arthritis and arthralgia as extraintestinal manifestations in patients with inflammatory bowel disease treated with vedolizumab: A meta-analysis. *Inflamm Bowel Dis.* 2023;29(Suppl 1):S1–2.

76. Nielsen OH, Munck LK. Drug insight: Aminosalicylates for the treatment of IBD. *Nat Clin Pract Gastroenterol Hepatol.* 2007;4(3):160–70.

77. Lim WC, Wang Y, MacDonald JK et al. Aminosalicylates for induction of remission or response in Crohn's disease. *Cochrane Database Syst Rev.* 2016;7(7):CD008870.

78. Akobeng AK, Zhang D, Gordon M et al. Oral 5-aminosalicylic acid for maintenance of medically-induced remission in Crohn's disease. *Cochrane Database Syst Rev.* 2016;9(9):CD003715.

79. Adwan MH. Drug Reaction with Eosinophilia and Systemic Symptoms (DRESS) syndrome and the rheumatologist. *Curr Rheumatol Rep.* 2017;19(1):3.

80. Cardones AR. Drug Reaction with Eosinophilia and Systemic Symptoms (DRESS) syndrome. *Clin Dermatol.* 2020;38(6):702–11.

81. Hama N, Abe R, Gibson A et al. Drug-Induced Hypersensitivity Syndrome (DIHS)/Drug Reaction with Eosinophilia and Systemic Symptoms (DRESS): Clinical features and pathogenesis. *J Allergy Clin Immunol Pract.* 2022;10(5):1155–67 e5.

82. Michel F, Navellou JC, Ferraud D et al. DRESS syndrome in a patient on sulfasalazine for rheumatoid arthritis. *Joint Bone Spine.* 2005;72(1):82–5.

83. Moya-Martinez C, Nunez-Hipolito L, Barrio-Gonzalez S et al. Azathioprine hypersensitivity syndrome: Report of two cases with cutaneous manifestations. *Clin Exp Dermatol.* 2021;46(6):1097–101.

84. Shiohara T, Mizukawa Y. Drug-induced Hypersensitivity Syndrome (DiHS)/Drug Reaction with Eosinophilia and Systemic Symptoms (DRESS): An update in 2019. *Allergol Int.* 2019;68(3):301–8.

85. Aota N, Hirahara K, Kano Y et al. Systemic lupus erythematosus presenting with Kikuchi-Fujimoto's disease as a long-term sequela of drug-induced hypersensitivity syndrome: A possible role of Epstein-Barr virus reactivation. *Dermatol.* 2009;218(3):275–7.

86. Mizukawa Y, Aoyama Y, Takahashi H et al. Risk of progression to autoimmune disease in severe drug eruption: Risk factors and the factor-guided stratification. *J Invest Dermatol.* 2022;142(3 Pt B):960–8 e9.

87. Yiasemides E, Thom G. Azathioprine hypersensitivity presenting as a neutrophilic dermatosis in a man with ulcerative colitis. *Australas J Dermatol.* 2009;50(1):48–51.

88. Frank J, Fett N. Azathioprine hypersensitivity syndrome. *J Rheumatol.* 2017;44(12):1876–7.

89. Bidinger JJ, Sky K, Battafarano DF et al. The cutaneous and systemic manifestations of azathioprine hypersensitivity syndrome. *J Am Acad Dermatol.* 2011;65(1):184–91.

90. McKenzie PL, Chao Y, Pathak S et al. Azathioprine-induced hypersensitivity reaction mimicking sepsis in a patient with systemic lupus erythematosus. *Mod Rheumatol Case Rep.* 2023;7(1):74–7.

12

Future Synergy between Rheumatology and Gastroenterology

MAYA NOELLE FAISON AND REEM JAN

INTRODUCTION

Gastroenterological complaints touch every disease in rheumatology, and conversely, inflammatory joint, skin, and eye symptoms frequently complicate the care of patients with inflammatory bowel disease (IBD). This chapter will review the immunological intersection between these two disciplines and summarize how we can learn lessons from our patients to inform progress in both fields.

THE MICROBIOME AND RHEUMATIC DISEASE

The microbiome refers to the composition of microorganisms, including bacteria, fungi, and protozoa, that can be found in locations like the mouth, GI tract, skin, and vagina (1). In this chapter, the term "microbiome" will specifically refer to the gut microbiome.

Research has demonstrated that the microbiome influences the immune system, including B cell– and T cell–mediated responses (1). Dysbiosis, or changes in the microbiome, has been implicated in multiple chronic diseases including obesity, type 2 diabetes, and even inflammatory and autoimmune conditions (2). As expected, the microbiome of patients with rheumatic diseases, including rheumatoid arthritis (RA), spondyloarthropathy, and systemic lupus erythematosus (SLE), has been studied and shows significant dysbiosis when compared to healthy controls.

In a recent systematic review, patients with RA demonstrated increased species of *Prevotella* and *Lactobacillus* along with decreased species of *Bacteroides* and *Hemophilus* (3). In another review, *Faecalibacterium*, which is postulated to have anti-inflammatory effects and assist with maintenance of gut homeostasis and permeability, was decreased in patients with RA (4). Within RA-related microbiome research, patients are often classified by stage of disease with comparison between pre-RA, early-RA, or new-onset RA, and patients with longer-standing diagnoses. Dysbiosis has been demonstrated, even for patients with pre-RA, which strengthens the hypothesis that dysbiosis plays an important role in RA development (5).

Similar to RA, patients with spondyloarthritis have significant differences in the makeup of their microbiome. It has been shown that spondyloarthritis patients have increased species of *Proteobacteria*, *Enterobacteriaceae*, and *Bacteriodaceae* with decreased species of *Bacteriodetes*, *Bacteriodales*, and *Akkermansia* (6). HLA-B27 is a genetic variance commonly associated with spondyloarthritis. While HLA-B27 is associated with dysbiosis, these changes do not always align with the general microbiome changes seen in spondyloarthritis patients, which presents an area for future research (6).

In patients with SLE, two studies have demonstrated increase in *Proteobacteria* and decrease in *Firmicutes*. However, this was not also demonstrated in a third study examined in a systematic

DOI: 10.1201/9781003367307-12

review (7). Interestingly, patients with active SLE and lupus nephritis show increased prevalence of *Ruminococcus* gnavus (8). This suggests that the microbiome may play an important role in lupus activity and disease manifestations, like lupus nephritis.

MANIPULATION OF THE MICROBIOME: DOES IT HELP?

Correcting the dysbiosis of patients with rheumatic disease represents a possible adjunct treatment strategy. The most commonly proposed and studied mechanisms to correct dysbiosis include probiotics and fecal transfer. It should be acknowledged that dietary change, like the addition of fermented foods, is also an area of interest but will not be discussed in depth in this chapter.

Overall, studies of probiotics show mixed results (9). Promisingly, a randomized control trial of 60 patients with RA taking *Lactobacillus acidophilus, Lactobacillus casei,* and *Bifidobacterium bifidum* demonstrated significantly lower disease activity, as represented by DAS-28 scores, and c-reactive protein levels at 8 weeks (10).

Similarly, fecal transplants have a conflicting body of research. In a randomized trial of 30 patients with psoriatic arthritis, patients treated with fecal transplant had significantly higher rates of treatment failure, defined as needing a step-up in therapy, when compared to placebo (11). Conversely, in a single-arm trial of 20 patients with SLE, there was significant improvement in disease severity, measured by SLEDECAI-2K scores, and anti-dsDNA at the 12-week endpoint (12). While encouraging, the lack of a placebo control arm in this trial presents challenges to its interpretation.

FUTURE DIRECTIONS FOR THE MICROBIOME IN RHEUMATOLOGY

The microbiome presents an exciting and complex area of future inquiry in rheumatology and gastroenterology. Research into the microbiome and dysbiosis raises important questions about monitoring and treatment of rheumatic disease. Future work is needed to elucidate if improved disease control in rheumatic disease reliably correlates with return toward typical microbiota. If this is the case, the microbiome could be utilized as an additional measure of disease control. This could be

especially useful for patients with rheumatic disease in its earliest stages, like pre-RA or early-RA.

Further research is also needed to understand the full clinical effect of adjunct therapies targeting the microbiome, including probiotics and fecal transplant. For probiotics, the impact of strain, dose, and dosage frequency are future areas of inquiry that could affect efficacy of therapy. For fecal transplants, further research is similarly required to understand the clinical effect of more frequent transplants and more varied transplant donors. For all treatments targeting dysbiosis, it may be useful to understand if larger changes in the microbiome toward normal flora correlate with greater efficacy of adjunct therapy to help provide treatment targets.

MOTILITY DISORDERS: NEW SOLUTIONS FOR A THORNY PROBLEM

If there is one common conundrum faced by rheumatology and gastroenterology in patients with connective tissue diseases, it would be the overarching theme of dysmotility. This can occur from esophagus to colon, and in scleroderma bowel disease, multiple sites may be involved at once. To date, these more extreme cases of ileus and colonic dysfunction have necessarily been managed by total parenteral nutrition.

A promising area of research focuses on the neuro-immunological drivers of autoimmune dysmotility. It has been postulated that autoantibodies targeting the ganglionic nicotinic acetylcholine receptor (gAChR) may mediate autoimmune enteric dysfunction (13). One study selected 39 patients with documented GI hypomotility and suspected autoimmunity based on co-existent autoimmune disease, family history, positive gAChR or clinical suspicion (14). Of these patients, 17 responded to a 4- to 12-week course of either IVIg or methylprednisolone. Twelve of these patients had neural specific autoantibodies, of whom six were gAChR. This study is interesting for a number of reasons. There were six other antibody types described in these patients, which highlights the need for a validated and comprehensive approach to serological screening for autoimmune enteric failure. Only one patient had an underlying rheumatic disease (lupus), and so the ability to extrapolate to all rheumatic patients is limited.

However, there can at least be an argument that the presentation of additional discernible signs of autoimmune nervous system dysfunction should prompt further workup in patients with connective tissue disease. Research is required to better define these autoantibodies and their relevance in patients with Sjogren's, lupus, and systemic sclerosis.

Gastroparesis remains difficult to treat in all patients, and in patients with systemic sclerosis, the etiology may be mechanical rather than immune mediated. There has been no role demonstrated for immunosuppression for the GI manifestations of scleroderma (15). Where prokinetics and dietary modifications fail to alleviate symptoms, gastric pacemakers have been tried for gastroparesis. While we could find no reports of their use in scleroderma, there is one series of 17 patients who underwent transcutaneous electrical nerve stimulation (TENS) of GI acupuncture sites for 2 weeks, with improvement in abdominal pain and bloating (16). There seems to be potential to explore these types of mechanical interventions further. However, the more frequent challenge in scleroderma is bowel hypomotility, for which no adequate solution is available.

EXTRAINTESTINAL MANIFESTATION OF INFLAMMATORY BOWEL DISEASE: THE NEXT FRONTIER

The arthritis associated with inflammatory bowel disease has long been a neglected area of rheumatology, with most of the management data extrapolated from psoriatic arthritis and axial SpA. However, there may be disease characteristics unique to this population that merit consideration of separate study.

Most of the clinical data for IBD arthritis comes from database reviews. As we have seen in previous chapters, the peripheral subtypes can vary from a spondyloarthritis pattern with large-joint involvement, enthesitis, and dactylitis to a more chronic symmetric small-joint arthropathy. Axial disease mirrors the clinical characteristics and imaging findings of ankylosing spondylarthritis but with some key differences. There is a high rate of asymptomatic sacroiliitis found on imaging studies of patients with IBD; this has been described on both CT abdomen and MR enterography (17, 18).

The natural history of these patients is unknown; prospective studies are required to define which of these patients will develop clinically meaningful axial disease. This has treatment implications, as the biologic therapies that treat IBD and that target axial SpA do not perfectly overlap (Figure 12.1).

There are also discrepancies in the literature on exactly how common or clinically meaningful IBD arthritis is. In terms of prevalence, peripheral arthritis appears to be the most frequent finding (13%), followed by sacroiliitis (10%) (19). This same systematic review and meta-analysis that examined 71 studies notes that few estimates were available for enthesitis (prevalence range from 1% to 54%) and dactylitis (prevalence range from 0% to 6%0. However, a more recent systemic review of the literature interrogated the study design of many of the IBD arthritis studies and found them wanting (20). For example, most of the 69 included studies were single center (68%). In 38 studies that evaluated axial disease in prospectively enrolled patients, inflammatory back pain was analyzed in 53%. SpA classification criteria were used in 68%, and imaging was performed in 76%. In 35 studies that evaluated peripheral disease in prospectively enrolled patients, SpA classification criteria were used in only 46%. A physical exam was performed in 74%, but of these patients, only 54% of them had an exam performed by a rheumatologist.

There is so much to be gained from improving our understanding of arthritis in patients with IBD. Beyond the clinical characteristics of these patients, there may be pathophysiological variances between patients with gut-limited disease and those with extraintestinal manifestations. One recent study looked at biomarkers of collagen degradation in healthy controls (HCs) and in patients with axSpA, CD, and CD-axSpA overlap (21). C4M, a fragment of MMP-mediated type IV collagen, found in the basement membrane, has been shown to be upregulated in axSpA and to have potential as a biomarker of treatment response in CD. This study showed that degradation of type IV collagen quantified by C4M showed a complete separation of patients with CD-axSpA overlap, compared to axSpA, CD, and HCs, and indicates excessive collagen degradation and epithelial turnover in this group.

What experience teaches us is that the presence of arthritis may lead to increased disability, healthcare utilization, change in IBD therapies, and

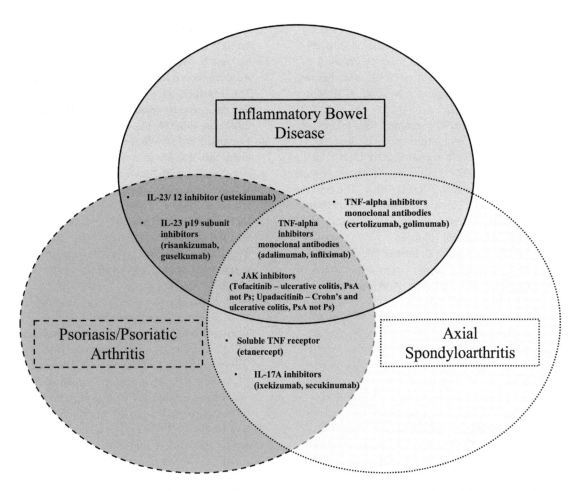

Figure 12.1 The disparate effectiveness of approved biologics for inflammatory bowel disease, psoriasis, and axial spondyloarthritis.

higher rate of combination DMARD or biologic therapies. Further studies, however, are required to prove whether these clinical impressions are in fact consistent and true. There are research consortiums being formed between multiple US centers that include both rheumatologists and gastroenterologist, and these types of initiatives may better identify and describe patients with IBD and joint pain to allow for such research questions to be answered.

CONCLUSION

Increased research collaboration between rheumatology and gastroenterology is an essential strategy to improve our care for patients with rheumatic disease who develop GI complaints and complications. These patients also provide a rich resource for gastroenterology to improve in understanding and treatment of motility disorders, which are highly prevalent and often severe. The relationship between the microbiome and the immune system is complex, and patients with rheumatic disease supply the scientific world with the ideal opportunity to elucidate these pathways. Finally, inflammatory bowel disease–associated arthritis provides learning opportunities for both specialties on the pathophysiology, clinical characteristics, and outcomes of these patients and a unique opportunity for drug development to target multisystem immune dysregulation.

REFERENCES

1. Pickard JM, Zeng MY, Caruso R et al. Gut microbiota: Role in pathogen colonization,

immune responses, and inflammatory disease. *Immunol Rev.* 2017 Sep;279(1):70–89.

2. Clemente JC, Ursell LK, Parfrey LW et al. The impact of the gut microbiota on human health: An integrative view. *Cell.* 2012 Mar 16;148(6):1258–70.

3. Bergot AS, Giri R, Thomas R. The microbiome and rheumatoid arthritis. *Best Pract Res Clin Rheumatol.* 2019 Dec 1;33(6):101497.

4. Chu XJ, Cao NW, Zhou HY et al. The oral and gut microbiome in rheumatoid arthritis patients: A systematic review. *Rheumatol.* 2021 Mar 1;60(3):1054–66.

5. Alpizar-Rodriguez D, Lesker TR, Gronow A et al. Prevotella copri in individuals at risk for rheumatoid arthritis. *Ann Rheum Dis.* 2019 May 1;78(5):590–3.

6. Wang L, Wang Y, Zhang P et al. Gut microbiota changes in patients with spondyloarthritis: A systematic review. *Semin Arthritis Rheum.* 2022 Feb 1;52:151925. WB Saunders.

7. Silverman GJ, Azzouz DF, Alekseyenko AV. Systemic lupus erythematosus and dysbiosis in the microbiome: Cause or effect or both? *Curr Opin Immunol.* 2019 Dec 1;61:80–5.

8. Azzouz D, Omarbekova A, Heguy A et al. Lupus nephritis is linked to disease-activity associated expansions and immunity to a gut commensal. *Ann Rheum Dis.* 2019 Jul 1;78(7):947–56.

9. Ferro M, Charneca S, Dourado E et al. Probiotic supplementation for rheumatoid arthritis: A promising adjuvant therapy in the gut microbiome era. *Front Pharmacol.* 2021 Jul 23;12:711788.

10. Zamani B, Golkar HR, Farshbaf S et al. Clinical and metabolic response to probiotic supplementation in patients with rheumatoid arthritis: A randomized, double-blind, placebo-controlled trial. *Int J Rheum Dis.* 2016 Sep;19(9):869–79.

11. Kragsnaes MS, Kjeldsen J, Horn HC et al. Safety and efficacy of faecal microbiota transplantation for active peripheral psoriatic arthritis: An exploratory randomised placebo-controlled trial. *Ann Rheum Dis.* 2021 Sep 1;80(9):1158–67.

12. Huang C, Yi P, Zhu M et al. Safety and efficacy of fecal microbiota transplantation for treatment of systemic lupus erythematosus: An EXPLORER trial. *J Autoimmun.* 2022 Jun 1;130:102844.

13. Nakane S, Mukaino A, Ihara E et al. Autoimmune gastrointestinal dysmotility: The interface between clinical immunology and neurogastroenterology. *Immunol Med.* 2021 Jun;44(2):74–85. PMID: 32715927

14. Flanagan EP, Saito YA, Lennon VA et al. Immunotherapy trial as diagnostic test in evaluating patients with presumed autoimmune gastrointestinal dysmotility. *Neurogastroenterol Motil.* 2014;26(9):1285–97.

15. McMahan ZH, Kulkarni S, Chen J et al. Systemic sclerosis gastrointestinal dysmotility: Risk factors, pathophysiology, diagnosis and management. *Nat Rev Rheumatol.* 2023 Mar;19(3):166–81.

16. McNearney TA, Sallam HS, Hunnicutt SE et al. Prolonged treatment with Transcutaneous Electrical Nerve Stimulation (TENS) modulates neuro-gastric motility and plasma levels of Vasoactive Intestinal Peptide (VIP), motilin and Interleukin-6 (IL-6) in systemic sclerosis. *Clin Exp Rheumatol.* 2013 Mar–Apr;31(2 Suppl 76):140–50.

17. Chan J, Sari I, Salonen D et al. Prevalence of sacroiliitis in inflammatory bowel disease using a standardized computed tomography scoring system. *Arthritis Care Res* (Hoboken). 2018 May;70(5):807–10.

18. Gotler J, Amitai MM, Lidar M et al. Utilizing MR enterography for detection of sacroiliitis in patients with inflammatory bowel disease. *J Magn Reson Imaging.* 2015 Jul;42(1):121–7.

19. Karreman MC, Luime JJ, Hazes JMW et al. The prevalence and incidence of axial and peripheral spondyloarthritis in inflammatory bowel disease: A systematic review and meta-analysis. *J Crohns Colitis.* 2017 May 1;11(5):631–42.

20. Schwartzman M, Ermann J, Kuhn KA et al. Spondyloarthritis in inflammatory bowel disease cohorts: Systematic literature review and critical appraisal of study designs. *RMD Open.* 2022 Jan;8(1):e001777.

21. Nielsen SH, Stahly A, Regner EH et al. Novel biomarker of collagen degradation can identify patients affected with both axial spondyloarthritis and Crohn disease. *J Rheumatol.* 2022 Dec;49(12):1335–40.

Index